Survival of the Spirit:

My Detour Through a Retirement Home

Ruth Howard Gray

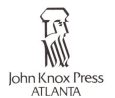

John Knox Press
ATLANTA

Acknowledgment is made to Alfred A. Knopf, Inc. for permission to reprint from page 201 of Dag Hammarskjold's *Markings*, translated by Leif Sjoberg and W. H. Auden. Translation copyright © 1964 by Alfred A. Knopf, Inc. and Faber and Faber, Ltd. Foreword copyright © 1964 by W. H. Auden. First printed October 15, 1964. Originally published in Swedish as *Vägmärken*. © Albert Bonniers Forgal AB 1963.

Library of Congress Cataloging in Publication Data

Gray, Ruth Howard, 1894–
  Survival of the spirit

  1. Gray, Ruth Howard, 1894– . 2. Aged—
United States—Biography. 3. Retirement—United States—
Case studies. 4. Old age homes—United States—Case
studies. I. Title.
HQ1064.U5G68 1985   362.6'1   85-42823
ISBN 0-8042-0911-1 (pbk.)

Contents

Dedication
To Doctor Robert Franch,
My physician and good friend.

Foreword

When she arrived at the retirement home at the age of eighty-five, Ruth Gray was prepared to make some adjustments but not to surrender abjectly to all the rigidities of the institutionalized care of the aged that confronted her now. What the staff called orientation looked to her suspiciously like a process of breaking in, or maybe breaking down, and she was not ready to be broken. She did walk with a cane and wear a hearing aid, to be sure, but she retained her capacity to think and evaluate, and this she intended to exercise. In order to "keep things clear" in her mind she began to jot down her reactions to life in an institution for the elderly, but she was not sure what she would do with her jottings.

This book really got underway when a twisted knee put her in the hospital. Ruth says now that her aged ego had suffered more damage than her arthritic knee. Both of her doctors sensed that. She told her arthritis doctor of the writing she was doing, and he encouraged her to continue. Doctors need to learn much more about treatment of the aged, he told her, and he would like to read what she wrote. Later on the same day she told her heart doctor about her jottings. He was even more enthusiastic and offered to help with typing the manuscript.

From that moment Ruth was committed to her project. She would have to do it to save herself. All around her people were saving themselves by submitting to the expectations of those who assumed they knew what was best for old people. They had woven for themselves a cocoon from which they did not expect to emerge as a butterfly. They were saving themselves by conforming. Ruth would save herself by recording the story of her rebellion.

Her whole life had prepared her for writing this book. Her father was a member of the founding faculty of a major school of theology and the second pastor of the church on that school's university campus. Reared in a parsonage and later married to a minister she understood well the caring work of the pastor and assumed that work as her own. In a later generation she might herself have sought ordination.

The great Christian education movement was challenging the younger leaders of the southern churches as Ruth reached maturity, and here she found a field in which to develop her interests and respond to her calling. She set about acquiring competence in the Christian education of children and soon was widely sought as a teacher and resource person in leadership courses, workshops, and laboratory schools throughout her denomination. When in 1949 she came to the staff of a large city church, she was the first Director of Children's Work in the city. While there she set up that church's weekday kindergarten, which became a model for many others in the Southeast. Meanwhile, she began writing poetry and stories for children, contributing articles to professional magazines, and preparing curriculum materials for the denomination.

Ruth Gray's life was devoted to children and the teachers of children. She wanted teachers and parents to understand how children feel, how they defend themselves, and what institutions do to them. She was firm in probing unexamined assumptions about what was good for children. Occasionally, ministers and church school leaders took offense at her persistent advocacy of the children's cause, but far greater in number were those of her generation who thanked her for the new sensitivities she nurtured in them. However today's pedagogical theories may differ from those she espoused, the fruits of her advocacy are still being harvested.

She had an enviable capacity to explore interests with others and grow along with them. Her interests in art, music, and literature spilled over into her own family and all her work with children. One of the strongest formative influences in her life was her relation to her sister, a victim of cerebral palsy. Her guidance, encouragement, and spiritual nurture was a determinative factor in the sister's pioneering work in the education of the brain-damaged. This relationship engendered in Ruth a passionate concern for the handicapped many years before that concern gained priority on the agendas of churches and schools.

Hardly a crusader, Ruth was yet confident in her faith. Her faith, shaped generally by the liberal theism of the early twentieth century, was nourished by a warm devotional life which flowed out of her immediate experiences of God and her love for all of God's creation. She was patient with conservatism and fundamentalism unless and until they became covers for exploitation. She had no use for pious posturing, and she punctured it with gentle humor.

To one who has known her the Ruth Gray portrayed on these pages is in character. By her own testimony she is now "the very same Me as the babe I was born—plus eighty-five years of living." One who had spoken so often in behalf of the children is qualified now to speak for the elderly and especially for those who because of fear cannot risk speaking for themselves. She wants people to know how old people feel, how they protect themselves, and what well-intentioned programs and institutions do to them. Her bathroom becomes a symbol of the grotesque arrangements often made for older people. She wagers that the toilet was designed by an able-bodied forty-year-old man.

It is such humor that makes Ruth's story so thoroughly delightful—and enables her to survive. It stands in contrast to a laughter-less environment. She hears very little laughter save when entertainment is brought in from the outside. People are free neither to laugh nor to cry.

This brings us to Mr. Brown, the shy widower who moves

into the apartment next to Ruth's. Had she not already known him she would have been drawn to him by his ability to laugh. She estimated that laughter increased tenfold after his arrival. His hassles with the maintenance staff and the maneuvering to get seated in the dining room are memorable episodes. His knack for gathering intelligence makes us all his debtors. He is Ruth's ally and fellow rebel, and his decision to leave the home hastens her own departure. Her simple and poignant narrative of the circumstances of his death was for me the most compelling part of her story. Death has never been so very far away, and here she lets us meet it.

I visited Ruth—she was eighty-eight then—in the home she had found where the Spanish moss trails from the oak trees. I called from my motel, and she came to fetch me in her car. We spoke of persons we both loved, and she told me more about Mr. Brown. We laughed together.

—Dr. James W. May

In the Beginning

Preview

I have arrived. Not trailing clouds of glory, not with any fanfare of greeting, but via a most ordinary vehicle: eighty-five years of aging.

I am a very important person, much in the public eye and press. I have many titles: Senior Citizen, Golden Ager, Retiree, Elderly. (There are three stages of elderly: elderly, middle elderly, elder elderly.) Some even call me and my peers the Old Folks, or Oldsters. The under-sixties (the dears), especially enjoy coming up with new names or phrases.

What it all boils down to is that we have become specimens, living in invisible test tubes. Scientists, the medical world, educators, sociologists, religionists (I use the term broadly), and the everyday person on the street all have a go at us. Put a little red in the tube today, a little blue tomorrow, shake well, let it settle, and see what you get. Almost a new race, or a new species of the evolving human being. Just imagine living to be ninety or over and still able to function, with limitations! We are truly an intriguing lot.

But enough of that. I said I have arrived, and I have: at a definite point in time and space. In the fall of the year and the winter of my life I have come to a "rest" home—rather, a "retire-ment" home, run by my own denomination. Age eighty-five, fe-male, still on two feet though walking with a cane, eyesight very good, deaf to the point of needing a hearing aid, hair not very gray and still thick, health very good except for arthritis, I still have the mental capacity to think, feel, and evaluate my reactions as I enter and live in this retirement home. I shall report it like it is—good, bad, and indifferent.

Monday. I arrive for a two-day visit in the company of my daugh-ter—not with fear and trembling, for I have been here before. I have friends here. It is a beautiful place, set in a valley with a stream meandering through the grounds. There are bridges over the stream, seats here and there. One could not wish for a better view. Nature has been kind, and humans have added small garden plots of flowers.

My daughter has to leave immediately for an appointment, but I am warmly greeted by Mrs. Gordon, one of several residents who volunteer to help prospective residents get acquainted with the facilities. After this, if I wish to live here I may return—if the estab-lishment "passes" me. I do not have much baggage, only a small suitcase and a paper bag of three heavy books. I cannot carry much due to severe arthritis in my hands and wrists, and given a choice of clothes or books, I prefer books.

We go to the desk in the lobby to get the key to the guest room. As we turn away, I look for an attendant to take my bag. Seeing no one, I ask my hostess if there is someone to help. "No," she says in a polite voice with a few ice cubes thrown in, "we wait on ourselves here." I struggle to the elevator with my heavy books under one arm and holding my cane in my other hand. Mrs. Gor-don carries my suitcase.

At my door she hands me the key and also a handbook. "Please read the book, every word of it, before you leave," she says crisply. "I will return at 4:30 to take you down to dinner. The dining room opens at 4:45."

Imagine! "Do we have to go so early?" I almost gasp. I rarely eat before six.

"High school students serve dinner," she replies. "They arrive soon after three and want to leave on the 6:30 bus."

I held my tongue, but silently I asked, "Is the dining room for residents, or the help?"

I have an hour free. Since I have not come prepared to dress again I survey the handbook—a very good introduction to the home. I scan the index and turn first to the section headed "Religion in the Home." I see that we have no Sunday morning service here, but my church sends a bus each week. Sunday evening vespers, Monday morning devotions, and a Friday Bible study are all offered.

Next I look at the food section. Breakfast and lunch are cafeteria-style; dinner is served. The hours are much earlier than I am accustomed to: breakfast 7 to 8:30; lunch 11:30 to 1; dinner 4:45 to 6. The book says, "At dinner sit four to a table to be served. Please stagger the times you come to eat. If residents come at fifteen-minute intervals the service will be faster for everyone."

Along about the fourth page of the book is a letter of welcome beginning, "Some suggestions which may help you in starting this new way of life." I do not care to start *a new way of life* any more than I can help. I like my old way. But I have no objection to change if the change is better and more pleasant.

Later I felt somewhat grumpy when I arrived at the dining room— I wasn't yet hungry. However, the meal was very good and I managed to smile and be polite. I was left back at my door at six o'clock. My hostess remarked that I might like to watch television and reminded me to read the book, that it would take some time to read. I looked at the news and glanced at the book again.

At my second reading my eye was sharp for the way things are stated. I have already found one discrepancy: people do not stagger the times they go to the dining room. I now plan to visit a friend, look at television, then read until midnight. This is my usual way of life.

Tuesday. Already my life has begun to change. I got up at seven to be ready for breakfast at seven-thirty. This was really a terrific effort.

I hate to dress before I've had at least one cup of coffee, which is rarely before nine. I tried to appear wide awake, alert, and interested.

After breakfast we toured the building: the library, laundry, and working facilities, all of which I've seen before when visiting friends. But it was the duty of my hostess to show me everything. This home offers excellent services—more than most, perhaps.

After lunch I had a good nap and changed my blouse for a nicer one but wore the same pants. I was not informed before I came that it is customary to dress for dinner. At four-thirty I took an elevator to the ground floor. There are only two elevators, one of which is also used as a freight elevator (though not at meal times). In a twelve-story building it takes a good bit of going up and down to get two hundred people down for meals!

Just outside the elevator on the ground floor is a small open space, then a hall to the dining room. This hall, about nine feet wide, is called "the gallery." The left wall is entirely glass, with a beautiful view. On the right wall hang pictures which are loaned by artists or friends of the Home for residents to enjoy.

"The gallery is a place of rendezvous," my hostess said. It seems to me that very few people at a time can take advantage of it. Immediately inside are two sofas, each seating only three people. Their seats are very old and hard and slant to the back, so very few people here can get up from them without help. After a short distance are two chairs, then some large ferns, then four more chairs—two with openwork iron seats that look uncomfortable and two with very thin cushions. Beyond these is a bench with cushions, but no back. Only four people can sit together in any of these seats. Since the chairs are in straight rows and many people are deaf in varying degrees, I think communication must be limited.

The last half of the gallery on the glassed-in side has twelve rows of two chairs each, all facing the dining room door, like an old fashioned street car. These chairs, too, are openwork metal but do have thin cushions. "Some people come thirty minutes before each meal," said a friend who lives here. "Seats fill up with the same people, who seem to have an unwritten lease on a certain chair. One lady always leaves a piece of Kleenex in what she considers 'her' chair to be sure to claim it next time."

As each elevator unloads, a procession begins to form. Some people pause to speak to those in the chairs. A few people walk briskly, passing others, eyes straight ahead. Many use a cane. Some limp, some drag along, some take a friend's arm.

The dining room doors open. Those nearest all but fall in, a mixture of slow getter-uppers from the seats and fast walkers from the elevators. I wanted to hear the "Triumphal March" from *Aida*!

Wednesday. My visit is over. I've decided I'll come to stay. I don't like eating with a lot of chattering people, but everything considered, I feel it is the best thing to do. I have been ideally situated where I am, but now that I can no longer keep house because of arthritis, it is time to change. I've lived long enough to know life is made of choices, and there are no perfect places. At eighty-five one should not quibble.

Before I left, the Assistant Administrator invited me in for an interview. After asking the usual questions she began to probe my inner feelings about being old. I told her I have read and heard a lot about old people no longer feeling needed, but I am very thankful *not* to be needed, to be free of responsibility, to be lazy. I said I know the world can get along fine without me. I have a happy, satisfying relationship with my children and grandchildren—we like to be together, but not all the time.

I was not answering according to the book. She asked what my plans for the future are, what activities I liked before and what I like to do now. I said, "I have no plans, for I have no future; I like to do just what happens to come along that suits me." She stopped then, and asked what I like about the Home. I told her. She also wanted to know what I do not like and, being a frank person, I told her that, too. I wonder if that was a mistake.

Now I must go home and get ready to move. I have myself well in hand. I will adjust!

Starting
a New Way of Life

I have moved in. All went well except for one unfortunate happening. Things are brought to the loading dock, taken to a freight elevator, down one floor to the basement, through the basement to the larger elevator, which is lined with carpeting so furniture won't get scratched. The movers then take it to your apartment, or *unit* as it is called. Shortly before four o'clock my son-in-law Jack brought my clothes, some lamps, and other things in his car. The maintenance man on duty showed him how to operate the freight elevator and left. He should have done the operating himself. Jack did not move his hand away quickly enough from the lever and his little finger was caught and severely mashed. He and my daughter ran through the basement and up to the front desk. He was given the proper papers, and they rushed to a nearby hospital emergency room. His finger was not broken but badly mashed. The Home paid the bill, of course. I happened to come down to the desk just as Jack got there. None of us was upset. I could tell that the staff was greatly relieved that we did not raise a ruckus about it.

Mrs. Gordon, the hostess who helped me during my visit, again met me at the door. She showed me more about the apartment set-up, cooking unit, heating and air conditioner, etc. I plan to begin cooking my meals tomorrow, as I had to bring things from my refrigerator and will not finish moving today. She said she would meet me at four-thirty and introduce me at dinner. This is normally done soon after most people have arrived to eat, while orders are being taken. I told her I was not sure I would be through at my apartment in time to make it. As it happened I was through, but I remained in my unit deliberately until five-thirty. A seed of rebellion is beginning to grow. I feel a bit like I did seventy years ago when I was fifteen and first entered a female college!

My second day here. The dining room almost overwhelms me. What bothers me most is being among so many old people all at once—the only young are the servers. Of course I am one of the old people, too, but I am determined not to be engulfed in the maelstrom. We sit four to a table. The dining room ceiling is low, and because many people are deaf and some refuse to wear hearing aids, conversation roars.

I had to be introduced tonight. Someone tapped a bell and all became quiet. Mrs. Gordon introduced me, then I stood, bowed, and smiled. At once the noise resumed. I was reminded of a barnyard of turkey gobblers.

A church youth group was coming to sing at seven. It was not yet six when I finished. Mrs. Gordon asked if I would like to attend. "No," I said, "I am tired from moving and want to get straightened out."

She hesitated. "I think when people go to the trouble of coming to entertain us, we should go."

I thought it best not to comment.

Settling in. After two nights my hostess dropped me, but Mrs. Evans, a friend I have known for years, has invited me to sit at her table for dinner. She happened to have a vacancy at her table, and I appreciate being asked. (We sit anywhere for breakfast and lunch, but have assigned seats for dinner.) The other two women are friendly and seem glad to have me. There is one drawback. Three of us are deaf, which makes conversation rather limited, especially when more than a hundred other voices are all but breaking the sound barrier. Sometimes I watch mouths moving, heads bobbing, and hands gesturing and hear only buzzing sounds. Would that we had captions, like silent movies!

I am settling in, but I am sure I disappoint some residents whom I knew before I came. I was asked to chair a committee—there are twenty. I declined, saying I wanted to rest and get used to the change before making any commitments. One person who knew of some of my many former activities remarked how good it is to have me here ready to go on doing things. I replied, "Oh, no, I did not come here to get into things but to get away from things." She's been rather cool to me since.

I can say, however, that I have been welcomed by many. People were considerate about not calling on a newcomer right away, but I have had offers of help such as "feel free to use my phone until yours is installed." They seem glad to have me here and speak of what a wonderful place I've come to. They have asked "Do you like it here?" and "Do you think you'll be happy here?" so often, however, that I wonder if they fear I won't. Some say "This is your *home* now," and I feel they want to add, "Please don't dare say there is anything you don't like about it." I usually say that I have moved less than a mile, that I have visited the Home many times, and that my move was not a big break, like going to another town. But I wonder if they think I'm not complimentary enough.

Why do I feel so strange? Since the fourth day here I have felt unlike my usual self, but I cannot put my finger on why. At first I thought I was just physically exhausted from moving. After all, I have not been well this past year and have been under great strain from illness in the family. The feeling persists, however, and I should be rested from moving by now.

Could I be having difficulty adjusting to my new schedule? Getting up in the mornings a little before eight to get to breakfast before the door closes is truly a hardship. I am eating all my meals an hour earlier than I was used to before I came. Today I tried going to all meals a little later—I barely got to dinner in time to get my order taken. But I am still lethargic.

I have plenty to do, getting my one-room unit organized for what I hope will be comfortable living. Yet I come into the room, turn on some music, and sit down. An almost complete inertia envelops me, physically and mentally. I seem powerless to combat it.

"I have plenty of time," I think, *"no cooking to do, no marketing to speak of, no cleaning, just make my bed and straighten a bit."* I sit and look out the window. I think, *"I should write some friends and tell them I've moved. No, not yet."* A button has come off a blouse. *"I should get out a needle and sew it on. No, not yet."* I've been wanting to call on other new people. *"No, not yet."*

This invisible, inexplicable thing grips me. All I seem to do is read or sit and look out the window. Fortunately I face a hillside full of trees. The pines are straight, tall, and green at the top. At this time of the year the other trees are bare, their branches making interesting designs and contours. What intrigues me most is watching long freight trains go by across the valley, as many as ten a day with a hundred and fifty cars. And what gorgeous sunsets we have had! I've watched them all.

Taking a second look around. It has taken me about three weeks to wake up from this state of stupor. I feel as if I were coming out from under a drug, as if I have been out of my body looking at myself. Now I look at the Home. Things are not as they first seemed.

The outside areas are beautifully landscaped. Just now they are bare, but in spring and summer flowers of many varieties bloom. In small plots here and there, residents may grow what they wish. One woman grows roses that would be the envy of any florist. For those who can walk, there are paved walkways and paths into the wooded areas. Those like me who cannot walk far, however, are not permitted a wheelchair, and there is not a single comfortable place to sit in the garden. Only a few stone benches, without backs, down near the stream.

A concrete patio runs the length of the gallery outside. It could be a shady and delightful place to socialize after dinner in fine weather, but there are only four double seats and ten chairs. They are all heavy to move and a friend tells me that the openwork iron of the seats soon begins to cut your legs. She said that when the weather gets fine, some bring cushions down with them so they can sit outside a while after dinner.

Getting outside, however, can be a problem. The only electrically operated doors are the entrance doors to the lobby. The glass doors leading from the gallery to the patio are much too heavy for one person to push unless she has unusually strong arms. This is also true of the glass doors leading to the music room where many stop off to watch the large color television after dinner.

Walking after dinner is the most acceptable thing here. You achieve status if you are a good walker. There are those who are not up to doing much who gallantly struggle on tired legs and weary feet to keep up an appearance, at least. One friend who is really not at all well told me that walking exhausts her. When I asked why she does it, she replied, "Everybody says you ought to walk." I cannot walk, and so I usually go to my unit.

For its size, my unit does very well. It is one room, on the seventh floor, with windows across the entire outside wall. All units are alike except for apartments in each corner of the building, which have a living room. In the one-room units our "kitchen" is a single appliance with two electric burners, a small sink, a small refrigerator, and a small storage space—enough for the little cooking we do.

However, although it's good to have a refrigerator, it sits below the cooking element so that its bottom shelf is nearly level with the floor. This is hard on the anatomy of a person over seventy. I can barely make it just to reach in and out for things. To clean it I have to sit on the floor (no mean accomplishment) and pull out the bottom shelf—all the exercise I need that day!

We have maid service once a week. The bathroom is well cleaned, my bed linen changed, and a vacuum is run over the floor—but not under the bed, not under anything. "Dusting" consists of dusting around things. We are responsible for cleaning our own cooking units.

The bathroom has a shower stall but no tub, which is all right with me. The stall is a nice size, plenty of room to turn in if you feel like turning and can do so without falling. There is no upright rod on either side of the shower opening, however, and inside, the provision against falling is inadequate. There is also a lightweight plastic chair, which is good to sit on. But although there is a rod to hold onto when you get up, in order to walk out of the shower you must let go of that rod and lean over to reach the towel rod beside the lavatory. The lavatory has a very adequate medicine chest above it, and another cabinet for towels is above the toilet.

I have never seen a more awkward toilet. It is a good make, and works well, but has no tank—just a handle in the wall about three inches long and three-fourths inch in diameter. To flush while sitting you must reach behind you and give a back-hand twist, an awkward and difficult thing to do. Even outside visitors notice how hard it is to flush. I don't know what left-handed people do, unless they get up, turn around and bend over. But there's no use complaining. It is as well grounded as a cannon.

There is a rod to the right of the toilet to help you rise, but it is put on the wall at a slant. The bottom is too low to be any help, the top is too high, and the rod itself is slick. I wonder why they didn't put bands of rubber along it, like walkers have, for gripping? I am willing to bet this bathroom was designed by an able-bodied forty-year-old man.

There is no intercom in the bathroom, either. The only intercom in the entire unit is in the main room near the bathroom door. It is simple to operate—you push a button or pull a chain to get a connection. It's good to have. I just hope that if I fall, I am able to move to it or happen to fall near it.

Patterns begin to emerge. We new people are being asked to take on positions of responsibility. Some have, most of them younger than I. (The average age here is eighty.) It is expected that we volunteer to be on a committee, and if we don't volunteer, we may be asked. I refused and sensed an invisible frown. Yet even some of the younger residents are tired of doing things. Most of us have been active in our communities and our churches all of our lives. Many of the activities here are worthwhile and some of the entertainment very good, but for a time I want to be free of responsibility—especially of doing things just to be doing. At times I feel I have come to a beehive. "Be busy" seems to be the motto.

We have all sorts of people here—some pleasant and some unpleasant, from places far and near. I believe the I.Q. level must be above average, for many hold Ph.D.s. We have a few couples and a few singles, but most of us are widowed. Since there are about six women to each man, the place can't help but be woman oriented. There is a beauty shop for women, but no barber shop for the men. Very few men attend large group meetings or go to entertainments. I sense that the men are lonelier and more at sea than the women. At the same time, if a man wants to marry, he has a number of choices.

A new man has recently been seated at a table with three women. I cannot see their table from where I sit, but my friend Edith can. She tells me that Mrs. Troy, the youngest, best-looking woman, sits across from him and manages to linger after dinner to walk out by his side. Sometimes one of their other tablemates will get on his other side and the three of them walk to the elevator together. Whether the other two women are also angling we don't know, for they are not as obvious as Mrs. Troy. Although the man is a first-comer for breakfast, she manages to arrive just as he does. I am amazed at her boldness, having grown up in days when a woman was more subtle.

The love game is as old as Time, but I am surprised at its manifestations among us oldsters. Is it faster because time is running out—a sort of "shoot straight from the shoulder, Sister, and fast, if you don't want to miss"? It would be funny, were it not so pathetic.

Something else that disturbs me is the matter of friendships. I met Edith and her friend Laura in a community gathering some months ago. When I told them of my plans to move into the Home, they were delighted and asked me to dinner here with them the next Sunday. We have always had much in common and enjoy being together. They welcomed me most cordially when I moved in and offered to do anything they could to help me get settled. But after that, they seemed distant except inside my apartment or inside one of theirs.

I asked Edith about it finally, and she said something that bothers me. She said that everyone here has certain special friends, perhaps of long standing, with whom they associate more than others. She said some of her old friends resent having their special friends take on newcomers and might get jealous if she took me on. She asked that in public places such as the dining room, hall, or lobby, I not pause often to chat—just come quietly to her room for visits. I do not understand. Does being loyal to old friends mean one cannot acquire new ones?

A "buddy" arrives. Mr. Brown, a long-time family friend, has moved into the unit next to mine. The last three years have been sad ones for him. His wife had a long bout with cancer. Since then he has lived alone and done his own housekeeping with only his faithful dog for company. He had no close neighbors. When his dog died, he decided to give up his house. I helped him look at several places, and when I decided to come here, he applied at the same time.

He is a friendly, outgoing person, and a rebel, like me. He has a great sense of humor, just naturally makes funny remarks, and is a good teller of jokes. We both laugh a lot. I dare say there has been more laughter here than there was before we came.

He and I are very close friends. Some argue that such friendship is not possible between a man and a woman, that sooner or later sex intrudes. Thus humanity short-changes relationships because we undervalue deeper aspects of friendship. There are several men here with whom I have much in common and with whom I would like to discuss current events, books, and such, but neither they nor I will risk it. I believe men and women need each other all through life, but petty attitudes deprive us of one another. I am delighted that Mr. Brown has arrived.

The angling began before he even got here. I mentioned that he was coming and when he would arrive. A friend told me there was a run on the beauty parlor that day! The second night Mr.

Brown was here he was asked by one of the anglers if he played bridge. He said no. She asked what games he did like. "I do not like to play games," he told her. Then she invited him to her apartment for a visit. Will he be caught?

As soon as Mr. Brown arrived, Edith also invited him to tea with her friend Julia and me. (Considering the smallness of our units, four makes a nice number for a small party or luncheon. If you don't have a car, it is not easy to get out for refreshments even for such small occasions.) Julia then invited the three of us to lunch, and we had a very good time. I took the next turn. Mr. Brown wanted to return the courtesies, but since his apartment is too crowded for comfort (he can't even shut his closet door), he was not sure what to do. I offered to prepare refreshments for him, but he thought that too much trouble for me. We finally settled on having us in my apartment for wine and cheese this evening before dinner, since a poor menu was listed on the bulletin board.

After dinner, Mr. Brown told me not to continue these parties. I think perhaps he thought people might begin to link his name and Julia's. I feel sure Julia is not interested in getting married and am sorry to give up our fun. Edith and Julia are good "laughers," a rarity in the Home.

A *most unpleasant incident*. Mr. Brown and I have wanted to eat dinner together, but although a vacancy occurred at my table, I did not think he would fit in. Mrs. Evans is very dignified, and he laughs and jokes a lot.

A few tables away a woman sat alone. Each night as I watched her, I wondered why. Finally I learned that she was in the hospital for several weeks and lost her place at her old table. It occurred to us that maybe we could join her. I decided to ask Edith how to tread softly in this matter new to me, the placement at tables.

Edith said we are not supposed to request where we sit except for a favored few like Mrs. Evans, who was one of the first people to enter the home. It seems that Mrs. Dudley, assistant to the food supervisor, is the arbiter of our fate in these matters. To prevent her from seating Mr. Brown where *she* chose rather than where we wanted, I must first get a gift for her, then between meals I should go to the dining room—after checking to see who was in the gallery. Edith mentioned a few people I should watch out for. If I saw them, I should wait until the coast was clear.

When I got there, I should knock on the kitchen door and ask to speak to Mrs. Dudley.

I bought a nice, moderately priced toilet article, wrapped it, and succeeded in gaining entrance to the dining room unobserved. I carried my gift in a little bag I use for taking books to and from the library. Mrs. Dudley came out and very coldly asked, "Yes?" I felt like I was in a bank asking for a loan.

"I am a newcomer," I said, "and just want to say thank you and give you this." I proffered my gift. "I also wish to ask you a favor." I explained that Mr. Brown and I wished to sit together and boldly suggested, "Since Mrs. White is alone at a table, perhaps we could sit there. Another man might also be placed there in time, for Mr. Brown." Then I waited. Would the banker turn down my request?

"I'll see if it can be arranged," she said, "but it is very difficult to seat people as they wish."

"I know," I said. By this time I was disgusted with the procedure. I would not have minded the gift if I could have offered it after my request. Since tips are not allowed here, people often give presents instead. However, this seemed like a bribe.

I made my way back without seeing any of the "wrong" people. But not only do I resent this manner of getting something done, I also resent the fact that a person with the status of assistant to the chef and supervisor of maids has so much authority concerning residents. She is certainly not our Hostess, although we should have one. Her duties are more kitchen than dining room.

I told Laura about it. She said it was that way before she came—she doesn't know why. "I think the hospitality committee should be in charge of seating," I said.

"Many things here are not as they should be," she replied, "but I enjoy being here too much to complain."

Later. The maneuver paid off. Mr. Brown and I are now assigned to the table with Mrs. White. I explained to my old tablemates tonight why I am leaving. I also told them I have enjoyed eating with them, and will miss them. They in turn said they are sorry to see me go, but I don't think Mrs. Evans really cares. I think she is disappointed in me because I have not gotten more into things. Unless I feel like it or know something is to my liking, I do not attend events such as a weekly night of music by outside groups, slide shows, or a variety of other programs. I told her when I first came that I did not come here to "get into things," but like my hostess, she answered, "I think when a group takes the trouble to come and entertain us, we should attend." I did not reply. I saw no need to argue the matter.

Another music group is coming tonight. Surely out of two hundred people they can get an audience. A program from Lincoln Center is on television. Not for a minute will I give up my freedom of choice!

These ashes are warm. A woman has been placed at our table. We are now a quartet, and a very harmonious one it turns out to be.

Not many women will tell their age, but I would guess Eva Dean to be in her early seventies—at any rate, at least ten years younger than I. She is not as pretty as Mrs. White, but good looking, nevertheless. Her general appearance is pleasing. She is not too particular about how she gets her outfits together, but her clothes are of good quality. She wears real jewelry, most of which is inherited. She's an intellectual, though does not look like my stereotype of one. She and her husband were professors at different universities. She is also the author of several books. I find her very stimulating. She has a wide range of interests and is undoubtedly an independent thinker.

She has not long been a widow. The Home is a temporary arrangement for her until she decides where she will settle. She is debating living in this city, where her husband taught before retiring, or the city of the university where she taught many years ago. She has many friends in both places and is often absent from dinner to be with friends. We visit each other in our units and sometimes enjoy television programs together that are of special interest for discussion. We do not always agree on the viewpoint expressed, but that is good. We stimulate each other. Eva is fast becoming my best friend here. I hope she does not settle elsewhere soon.

Edith is very interested in our foursome. She loves romance. Already twice-married and now in very poor health, she is not interested in marriage for herself. She greatly enjoys watching other people play the game, however. Now that Mr. Brown is seated between two of the most attractive women here, she has focused attention on our table and is all but gambling on which one will win. I just let her go on speculating.

Meanwhile, we four enjoy our present state. Mrs. White has four children, fourteen grandchildren, and several great-grandchildren living in many places. She is frequently called to come when someone is ill or to come to a wedding. A husband would be a hindrance to her.

Eva really needs someone to look after her. She has only one son and is somewhat helpless about handling finances and deciding where she will live. But she has a very active, creative mind and likes to visit about in different cities. It would be hard for her to find a suitable husband.

How about me? I do not need to be looked after. If I did, I have three children. Old age does have advantages. For me to be freed of responsibility for others and to be my own boss over my time and actions is most pleasant.

Does Mr. Brown need a wife? He can very well look after himself—he's done so for more than three years. He did not marry until he was forty and will never find anyone to take his wife's place, no matter how fine a woman might be. I could be mistaken, but I don't think he will ever consider a second step into matrimony.

We did have the first wedding since I came here just a few days ago. We had no sign of a romantic situation beforehand. One of the younger women who has been here only a few months moved out into a swank apartment nearby. She said she had a lot of furniture and couldn't manage in the limited space she had here. Mr. Norton, a man in his eighties who lost his wife several months ago, said he had decided to move into the same complex. No one had any idea there would be a wedding. They announced it after it was over, when he moved in with her.

We were surprised—partly because he is so much older and in such poor health. This week we heard both are quite ill with flu. Neither have relatives in the city, and so they called a maintenance man from here to come over and help them after hours. He got their groceries and whatever else they needed, and returned to the Home full of news. When word of their marriage *and* their illness reached the Home, there were some snickers—as if to say, "You see, sex in old age will just lead to trouble!"

As is to be expected, the old are just as curious as the young about the sex life of the old—that is, the specific biological functions of sex. Does the sex urge ever die? People my age grew up when sex was not discussed openly, so it is not easy for most of us to discuss it now. Those of us who do not have mates don't go around asking those who do about their sex life, nor do we ask each other if we miss our former sex life. I think the answers to such questions would be as varied as the people questioned. Sometimes in print I read a statement such as, "There is no reason to believe that sex cannot continue until very late in life, if people are still well and active." Happy thought.

We have one couple here who are a real delight to behold. These two people formerly lived near each other. Each had four children, and their families were good friends. After the children grew into adulthood, the families lost touch. Then two spouses died. The other two met again, married, and came here to live.

I don't know their exact ages—eighty at least. They have become quite feeble, but they seem so happy and content, walking hand in hand or the wife holding the man's arm—though never acting silly or sentimental. Often they are away visiting one of his or her children. We miss them when they are away and are always glad to have them back.

Romance is certainly possible for the elderly. Though most of us do not experience it to a great degree, we can at least partake of it vicariously. It's nice to know that though the fires of passion may burn low, warm ashes of romantic feeling still remain.

Something to laugh about. Some of us were gathered in the hall talking when Mrs. Lane, a jolly eighty-five, came along to tell us of something that had just occurred. We laughed so hard that some of us had to sit down.

Mrs. Lane said that she had been out for a walk. When she came upstairs, Mr. Judson (one of the men residents) came up on the elevator with her and did not get off at his floor. He got off with Mrs. Lane and, after hesitating, asked if she knew which apartment Mrs. Parks lives in. Mrs. Parks is so new that she doesn't yet have a phone or her apartment number listed. Apparently Mr. Judson had seen her in the dining hall and liked her looks. Also, he is just recovering from being dismissed by another woman. He must have decided on the direct approach.

Mrs. Lane led him to the door and knocked, while he stood behind her. When Mrs. Parks opened the door, Mrs. Lane said, "Mr. Judson wants to see you."

Mrs. Parks had on her housecoat and was barefooted. "Just a minute," she said, "until I get on some shoes." Then she shut the door, leaving poor Mr. Judson outside.

Mrs. Lane came on to our end of the hall and, seeing us gathered, stopped to tell us about it. We could still see Mr. Judson far down the hall, waiting. We began to chuckle.

Then Mr. Brown said, "Maybe Mr. Judson could take off his shoes and leave them outside, Japanese style. That way they could start right off playing footsie." We laughed harder.

One of the women said maybe Mrs. Parks wanted to get her toenails cut, that it had once been requested of *her* by a man. We laughed so hard we almost became rowdy.

That is the first time since I've been here that so many people have laughed so hard together. We may laugh gently at dinner, or during an entertainment, but rarely do we laugh like Santa Claus, whose little round belly shook like a bowl full of jelly. Our bellies are *big* and round, but they certainly shook that night. Very likely we could be called silly (if not senile!) because we laughed about an old woman closing the door and putting on her shoes before she would admit a male caller, but how we do need "good ole belly-busting" laughter.

My Spirit
Is Vexed

For Our Dining Pleasure

Five months have gone by now in my new "home." Most people have quit asking "Do you like it?" or "Are you happy here?" When someone does, I say that it is a good place to be when you come to need some of the services it provides. I cannot bring myself to lie and say I love it here.

In many ways I have adjusted. The dining room, however, still nettles me. I say *nettles* because it is rather like a nettle rash—hard to ignore, but it only makes it worse to scratch.

When I first came to visit, I said they should play the "Triumphal March" from *Aida* to herald dinner. Now I think it should be Chopin's "Funeral March." As soon as the doors are open, the front people press in. Servers (mostly girls) rush to tables with order sheets. Menus on the tables list six entrees, from which we choose one. Each server waits on five tables. To fill in our order sheets, she may kneel on the floor and write on the table, hold her serving tray between her knees as she bends over to write, or use the tray as a board to write on. Why can't they just have a pad like restaurants have?

I have been told the servers are not trained, but that is so obvious I did not need to be told. Why they are not trained, I do not know. They receive wages for their work.

When a server comes back with food for a table, her order sheets may be dangling from her tray, between her teeth, or in her pocket. She sets the tray of four servings on a nearby table to look at her lists, then hastily sets plates on the table. Next she begins to remove juice glasses, soup bowls, and salad saucers (salads are always served in very small saucers) with the rapidity of a professional juggler. She grabs here and there, races across and around, and dumps the dishes in a large, deep dishpan which sits under the small serving table. So far, no one has stepped into one of those dishpans, although I've come close to it when leaving early.

This same hurry-scurry goes on when our plate is removed. We have to be alert to be sure it isn't snatched away before we finish. Tonight a lady at the table next to mine was winding up her dinner with a glass of milk and some crackers when the paper mat was pulled from in front of her!

Three or four waitresses serve as coffee and tea crew. A bowl of ice sits on the sideboard from which coffee and tea are served, and one girl regularly picks up ice with her hands to put into glasses for iced tea. When they are serving, waitresses carry coffee in one hand and hot water for Sanka or tea in the other. Iced tea is served separately. Packages of Sanka, tea bags, and artificial sweetener are carried in three pockets of their smocks. We are supposed to reach into the pockets for what we want. You may reach for sweetener and come up with Sanka. Of course, the server *can* set the hot liquid on the table and help us, but our tables are so small that the pot must rest close to an elbow or lap. We prefer to grab.

Some nights after the meal is over, sugar bowls are emptied into a large bowl so they can be washed. One such night three of us late-comers watched as a server broke up large lumps of sugar with her bare hands, then wiped her hands down her smock.

Since there is no Hostess in the dining room, there is no one to prevent such behavior. It is not uncommon for a girl to carry a glass of juice on her tray and drink from it between tables she is serving or for another to eat from a bowl of cobbler at the coffee table while she watches for hands raised for services. And why, oh, why, did I have to turn my head one evening just as a waitress leaned down, took off her shoe, scratched her bare foot, and continued to clear a table?

The Administrator never eats dinner here. Today, evaluation sheets were sent out with many categories listed to be checked Satisfactory or Unsatisfactory. Comments could be added if we wished. At the top of the first page it stated that one did not have to sign one's name. Many people, especially newer ones, are not satisfied with the evening meal. I wrote three pages on the food service and signed my name. Will it do any good?

The dinner meal was very good when I first came and has been in years past when I visited friends here. In recent months, however, it has gone steadily downhill. Even long-time residents agree. High prices and a continuous rise in costs are their excuse for smaller portions and inferior quality, yet resident prices have been raised and most people would prefer to pay even more for better quality. Nobody expects it to be like home, but we expect more than we get.

If we have slaw, it measures half a cup. Broccoli is one spray, maybe two, mostly stalk. Fruit bar is old bread softened with canned fruit cocktail and half-baked (a sorry goo). Stewed tomatoes are ruined with cornstarch and sugar. A few times a week we have a good-sized portion of chicken or beef, but chicken and dumplings is mostly dumplings with four to six bites of chicken, and beef tips on noodles has little beef. If we ever got prime rib or a breast of chicken, it might cause a few strokes!

Sunday dinner, after the buses return us from our churches, is always the best meal of the week. Friday dinner is the poorest. One choice is always fish—poor quality and not enough for a cat. Another dish, "hamburger pie," defies description.

Lunch is very good. Served cafeteria-style, it offers a better selection, a large bowl of tossed salad from which we serve ourselves, and really good desserts. Breakfast is also good. At dinner, only the coffee is really excellent. The Administrator often eats lunch here, sometimes breakfast. Dinner? Never!

The only problem with cafeteria-style meals for elderly people is that the trays and dishes are extremely heavy—for durability, I suppose. There is no help available to carry them, nor is there help with stacking them in racks after use. It is hard for a woman my age with weak arms and knees to carry a heavy tray, bend over to put it on a low rack, or stretch to reach a high one.

The cafeteria is small, so items such as juice glasses and saucers of fruit are crowded. The first morning Mr. Brown was here, he reached for a saucer of prunes on the front row just as a server shoved a saucer on the back row. One saucer fell off, hitting the rail and spattering juice into Mr. Brown's face. Then it bounced off his shoe, spilled juice on his trousers on the way down, and finally hit the floor. We laughed and have joked about it from time to time since. But we can laugh only so often. . . .

Please dress for dinner. Since this started out as an elite type of Home, it has always been the custom to dress for dinner. Most of the women have many pretty dresses, pantsuits, scarves, shawls, and sweaters—some quite expensive—and accessories to go with them. Rarely does someone wear the same outfit two nights in a row, or wear at dinner what she wore to breakfast, even if it was lovely. At dinner, jewelry is also much in evidence—large, long earrings, two or three necklaces, a pin, perhaps bracelets. The men always wear coats and ties.

Perhaps dressing up is a recompense for stooped bodies, wrinkles, thinning hair, and faded skin. Well-coiffed hair and bright dresses are certainly to be preferred over dowdiness. Compare, however, the outfits of residents with those of servers. Our waitresses wear smocks over whatever they wear from school. The smock slips over the head and has two narrow ties on each side of the waist to tie it in place. Often one tie has come unsewn, and the smock falls about during serving. Sometimes they are not tied even though they have not come unsewn. Some hems have come down, and not been repaired. Any smock worn over a long-tailed shirt that hangs three inches lower over jeans or pants is really interesting to behold.

Some of the girls wear flowing dresses under their smocks so that they will be ready for dates after work. Other times they bring clothes to put on before their boyfriends get here. One night when some of us were late finishing dinner, we saw a girl bring out her change of clothes and shoes, put them on an eating table, then pick up a mirror and proceed to comb her hair in the dining room.

Tonight one of our few boy servers had a tear in his jeans running from the bottom of his hip pocket to the stride. It gaped open to show his underwear. Unappetizing, to say the least.

Because of the poor food and service, many people say they would be embarrassed to invite a guest to dinner. Steak houses, hamburger joints, and lower-priced restaurants have more pleasing service. Why, then, do we dress up so, to eat such ordinary food served in such a slipshod manner?

We expect improvement. Soon after the evaluation sheets had been scrutinized, notices were sent out that a new head of food service, a highly qualified person, had been employed. We could expect improvement. Now we sometimes have a thin slice of orange on top of the chicken or a red apple round on the side of our plates. It does give a touch of color but does nothing to improve the food. It makes me feel like a sick child whom someone is trying to entice to eat. In plain words, it is camouflage to make us oldsters think we are getting something when we are not.

The funny thing (and how thankful we are for a few funny things) is names given to menu items. A salad called "Hidden Jewels" consists of chunks of orange and green gelatin with powdered sugar sprinkled on. "Blushing Pear Salad" is a very small lettuce leaf and half a pear (the cheap, canned, hard variety), with a bit of pink jelly in the center. Mr. Brown said recently, "No wonder it blushes. Lots of other things, too, would do well to blush."

Out of Order—Again

It would seem that those of us who have come within the last year arrived just as the place got ready to fall apart.

This morning I went to do some laundry in the laundry room. One of the washing machines had an Out-of-Order sign on it. It's been there since I came. After I put my clothes in to wash, I went up to lunch. When I came back and was about a foot from my washer, I slipped. Enough water had leaked onto the floor to make it slick. Quickly I caught my balance and did not fall.

I held onto the machine as I took my clothes out and put them in a dryer. Then I went in search of someone from the domestic staff to tell about the leak. The first woman told me it was not her job to mop floors—I would have to find someone else. I told two more people, without success. Finally I went to the head of maintenance, and after he had consulted with two more people, the floor finally got mopped.

Maintenance here is unusually slow, it seems to me. When Mr. Brown applied for entrance he was shown an apartment that would be available in a month. The cooking unit was not working, but he was told that a new part had been ordered and the unit would soon be fixed. After he'd been in the apartment for several weeks, he inquired and was told the part hadn't come. After another interval he inquired again and was told the same thing. He's usually very patient, but his patience was beginning to wear thin. Since the cooking unit is part of the entire kitchen unit, he also had no refrigerator, which he missed even more. It's nice to have ice, cold drinks, sandwich makings, and snacks on hand. Finally he suggested to the administrator that he buy himself a small refrigerator, and that was agreed to. (He was getting a reduction in rent since he had no cooking unit.)

He continued to inquire at the office and at the maintenance department whether they had any idea when he could expect repairs. They always replied, "We don't know," or "We hope soon." I admire him for his patience. After all, the firm which makes these units is in this very city.

Finally, one day a few weeks ago, the part arrived. He was told the unit would be set up the following week. The day came. The sink, top cooking plates, refrigerator, and storage space were set into place. However, there were no handles for the faucets, no stopper for the sink, no drain pipe from the sink to the pipe below. In another week the stopper and handles arrived. In yet another week the pipe came for the drain—but no rubber gasket to put around it where it joined the sink. Mr. Brown still awaits use of his cooking unit.

If we need a part, maintenance invariably replies, "It has not come." If something needs repairing, "We're working on it"—with no visible results. Sometimes I feel as if Maintenance is a spectre and not human beings.

The night the electricity went out. Our fire alarm system seems to be adequate. The alarm sounds at intervals for fire drills and we act according to instructions. There was no plan, however, no set of instructions for the emergency a storm caused last night: the current went off and the elevators stopped.

We were almost through dinner. Many people had already gone to their rooms, but about fifty of us remained on first floor. Suddenly the lights went out. In a few minutes the hall and lobby lights began to glow dimly as an emergency generator provided a bit of power. Trucks and crews arrived from the power company and did all the things they do first, without result. Since this is a very wooded area, scouts then went about in the woods and discovered a large tree had fallen on our line. Getting equipment to the area presented a big problem.

Meanwhile, we who were stranded sat in the gallery, the music room, and lobby, or just milled about. We could have sat more comfortably in the dining room, but it was in total darkness. People who lived on lower floors climbed the stairs, but those with bad legs or hearts and those of us who lived higher expected the elevators to begin running at any time.

At first there was laughter and talk, although a few people were distraught. Then the Administrator came to tell us that a tree was on the line, and it might take all night to get it off. He said no word of comfort or cheer or that any help would be offered those who could not make it up the stairs. Immediately the hall buzzed with discussion of how many stairs one could actually make. There are fourteen steps to each floor. Of the ten people on my end of the seventh floor, eight walked up. Among them were weak knees, weak ankles, and bad hearts. I have such a bad knee I knew I could not make even one flight, and so I waited below. Mr. Brown also waited, saying he did not mind sitting up all night.

One quite elderly couple walked to the twelfth floor. No word of caution was given, no one seemed to know what else to do.

I sat for a while beside Mrs. Tucker, a very deaf, very old lady who could not quite comprehend what had happened. I spoke right into her ear and told her. "Will they get it fixed?" she asked over and over again. "Will we have to stay down here all night? What will we do?" I kept telling her not to worry, that we would take care of her. But she seemed only to have caught what the Administrator said about it possibly taking all night to fix the power. After about thirty minutes, I got up to stretch. Someone else took my place to listen to her sad refrain.

Next I sat by a woman who is in very poor health. She needed her medicine. She knew she would be ill if she sat up all night. I cast my eye about for possible "beds." There is one sofa in the music room, and someone said there are a few cots in the basement used for guests of residents. All the chairs on this floor have arms, but I thought that the thin cushions could be put on the floor for pallets.

I was not worried for myself, for my daughter lives nearby. They were out for the evening, but I thought I would sit up until midnight and then call them if necessary. Several people had already called their families and departed.

The current went off about five-thirty. At eight I inquired of a friend who has been here several years whether she thought any action would be taken. She said she did not know. We were both aghast at the indifference of the Administrator. He did nothing but stand at the window and look out at the truck lights flickering in the woods where the men were working. At her request, one young man who had remained on duty at the lobby desk did walk up and get some medicine for a woman who knew him well. However, he did not volunteer to do the same for anyone else.

Finally, about nine, the lights came on, but we were warned not to use the elevators yet. "Give the fuses time to see if they are really okay," the Power Company man told us.

When he gave the signal, the young man from the desk ran to open the elevator doors. We nearly fell in. I was near enough to make the first one.

We have, of course, discussed the incident all day today. There were no falls, apparently, among those who walked up. A few say that their legs or backs hurt, but most of us are now taking it casually. After all, we didn't have to wait all night. Yet I cannot help thinking, "Suppose we had? There could be another time." A few of us who are willing to speak out discussed bringing up the matter at the next association meeting. I doubt if we will, though—we probably would not get enough support from other residents for anything to be done. They might fear someone would think them physically weak or cowards. A committee might be appointed, of course, and give recommendations. Ultimately, however, the administration should take responsibility to see that a power failure doesn't put the elevators out of commission or that an emergency plan is ready to function.

I wonder how many doctors would advise people eighty and beyond to walk up almost two hundred concrete steps?

Two days later. I just heard that a woman who walked to the fifth floor during the power emergency has had a heart attack and is hospitalized. And *still* there is no plan to prevent another occurrence.

Repeat performance. Tomorrow is Mother's Day, so there is more coming and going than usual. About three o'clock a call came up from the desk saying an outside friend wanted to come up to see me, if convenient. I gladly agreed. After five minutes (the elevators are sometimes slow), I went out in the hall to meet her. The fire doors were closed and the elevators were not running. Yet there had been no alarm nor warning.

Some young people had walked up to see their grandmother. They did not know what had happened. I tried to call the desk. First there was no answer, then I got a busy signal for many more minutes. Finally I got an answer—and an explanation. A transformer had failed. The volunteer on duty had called the Power Company, but we should not expect things to be fixed quickly on Saturday. We again had to stay put, whether up or down. The power came on in an hour, but I never did learn who came to visit me.

When you are seven floors up with a bad knee, an hour is a very long time. A lot of frustration can build up in that time. Being frustrated, peeved, provoked, and upset about so many things gets me into a state of almost constant tension. I find it hard to relax and rest here—the only ones who do have woven about them a cocoon from which they shall not emerge as butterflies. And yet, no one will agree to form a group to consider what we might do. Many say that if such a group were formed, they might take part, but no one wants to commit until others do so.

Is it the aging process itself that makes people lose their determination to act or does the environment in which we live defeat us? I suppose it is both. Naturally when we arrive at eighty we are not as efficient either mentally or physically as we were at thirty. Therefore, I think the environment should be as helpful as possible. Would that society would heed the declaration Ulysses made to his aging father Laertes:

> Warm baths, good food, soft sleep and generous wine.
> These are the rights of age and should be thine.

Am I *Still* My Neighbor's Keeper?

We have few written rules here. It is the unwritten ones—and interpretations of some of the written ones—that bother me. For instance, there is the written statement that "one must be mentally and physically able to live without attendant care, be ambulatory without use of walker, to live in this Home." Sometime, somewhere, the idea developed that one must neither give nor receive help in carrying cafeteria trays. Occasionally, if someone has had a hand or eye operation, the custom is varied for a short time, but soon those people are struggling with their trays again. They are afraid that if they are helped they will be asked to leave.

Marianne, a new resident, told me the following story: a ninety-year-old woman had an eye operation and had to wear a patch over the eye for several weeks. Her other eye was not very good either. After having her meals sent to her unit for a few days (a very commendable service here), she came down to the dining room for dinner and, being unable to see her own table, sat down in a vacancy at Marianne's. Marianne cut up her meat for her and helped her out of the dining room.

The next morning they went to breakfast together, and Marianne helped the woman again—got coffee for her, carried her tray, and later put it on the stand. She also walked with her to the elevator.

The second morning, as Marianne put both trays on the stand, someone came up behind her and said quietly, "You are not supposed to help Mrs. Simpson." It was Mrs. Roberts, a good friend of Mrs. Simpson's.

"Why not?" Marianne inquired, surprised. "She certainly needs help just now."

"We are supposed to be able to care for ourselves here," Mrs. Roberts said firmly. "It's the rule." It is *not* the rule that we are not supposed to help one another, but that's the way the rule is interpreted.

If Marianne's story hit me like a splash of water, a conversation of my own hit me like a downpour. Soon after warning Marianne not to help Mrs. Simpson, Mrs. Roberts herself fell as she stepped from the elevator and broke her hip. Her operation went well, and she went to her daughter's to recuperate. When she had been with her daughter about a week, I called to see how she was doing. Her daughter reported that she was doing well. She had been using a walker and now was practicing walking with two sticks. Walkers are not permitted here, but since she soon would not need a walker at all, she hoped to avoid going to a nursing home and to come directly back here from her daughter's. She has lived in this Home for so long that it is truly "home" to her.

I went down at mail time and, as usual, saw people I wanted to talk with. One special friend of Mrs. Roberts asked if I had heard from her recently. I told her about my call, and she was delighted at the report. Just then a second friend of Mrs. Roberts came up. The first said to me, "Tell Mrs. Barton what you told me about Mrs. Roberts."

When I finished, Mrs. Barton said in her precise voice, "Mrs. Roberts will not be able to carry her tray."

Since Mrs. Roberts can have her meals sent up for a week or more, and then might fix her own breakfast in order not to have to buck the cafeteria line, Mrs. Barton's response astonished me. "Oh,

I'm sure Mrs. Roberts has friends who will be willing to carry her tray," I replied.

"But it's against the rules." She spoke very seriously.

"What rule?" I demanded.

"We are not supposed to have help carrying trays," she said firmly.

"Who says?"

"We are supposed to be self-sufficient. When we have rules, I think we should keep them."

"Well, if it's a question of keeping a rule or being kind, I'll break the rule," I declared. "It is not written that one must not help a friend." Then, feeling I was pushing too hard, I ended the conversation on a lighter note.

As we moved on our separate ways, I marveled at the hardness of the wall of the cocoon which sometimes enwraps the older-elderly. Do we no longer love each other? The people here are above average. Some are rich, most are affluent, educated, and well-traveled. All of us have been used to a comfortable way of life and to taking responsibility for the world. How can we now be so crass concerning others? The old are betrayed not only by younger people around them but also by each other.

For instance, this morning I was in a group discussing the use of walkers. Some said they thought people who have to have one for just a few weeks or months should be able to do so. Others said they would be in the way in the dining room and opposed their use. Those who opposed have never needed one.

Someone suggested that people returning from the hospital could use a wheelchair to come from their room to the dining room door. Both walkers and wheelchairs could remain outside the dining room. There are still more able-bodied than feeble ones, and though not everybody would be willing to help, some would.

The alternative is for one to go from the hospital to the next level of care in this complex. That means sharing a room with someone else and being very crowded, which is certainly not conducive to recovery. A person going to the next level of care might have to room with a senile person who has reverted to childish behavior and has to be locked in at night. It seems needless for residents to have to go from here to there and back again, especially following an ordeal. A retirement home should truly be a rest home. A few concessions should be made.

Few are, however. One of my grandsons visited me for a few hours recently. The gardens are lovely just now, and as we stood high up on the breezeway and overlooked them, he asked if there were wheelchairs available so he could take me for a stroll. I had to shake my head. The nursing home patients are often taken for rides, but residents of the Home must be "ambulatory." That means no wheelchairs—even for people who can walk fine inside but need assistance with long jaunts or who might easily trip on the grass of the garden. When, oh when, will those of us who are involved be able to make our voices heard about the rules that determine our lives?

The lonely among us. By this time I realize that after the first few weeks of effusive greeting, you are left strictly alone. I would never have thought that visiting would be so limited. I have seen more of the friends I knew before I came; I have made a few new friends who are worthwhile, but only five people who did not know me previously have visited me in my apartment. The ten people on my end of the hall are congenial. We keep up with one another on the way to the elevator and in the hall, and on cleaning days we may sit in chairs in the hall to chat, but we never visit inside our apartments. As there is no lounge for gathering in the building, I thought people would visit in their own places more often. Only a very few do. Some of the men call the apartments "cells."

One day several weeks ago I brought from my daughter's yard a large bunch of blue hydrangeas. As I passed through the lobby, the woman sitting at the desk remarked about how beautiful they were. She is younger than many residents, a pleasant person who smiles often. Her disabilities, if any, do not show. Perhaps she is here because she is alone. I have thought ever since I came, "I would like to know her and be friends with her." After I got to my room I thought, "Why didn't I give her one of these flowers?"

I waited until I knew she would be off-duty and back in her unit, and then I phoned. She was in. I said that if it was convenient,

I'd like to come up and visit a bit. I took one of the hydrangeas. She seemed pleased, and appreciated my sharing the flowers with her. We had a friendly chat and I remarked as I left, "Come see me sometime." She never has.

I also shared my flowers with another woman who is severely handicapped by Parkinson's disease. She is using strong medication, and told me once that only a few hours a day is she free from shaking. She uses those intervals to go to meals. She has to wear a neck brace that holds her neck stiff. She walks along to the dining room at a normal pace, but never turns her head to speak because she cannot turn it without turning her body. Her voice is so weak it is very difficult to understand her. I go to see her occasionally just before meal time when she is under the medication and able to talk a bit. I stay about five minutes. It is understood that she is able to be active for only a few hours at a time. We seem to communicate without much being said. She has family here, which is a blessing. I've never seen her with anyone when she is going to meals or getting her mail. I don't know if she has special friends or not. I've asked my friends about her, but they do not visit her. Everyone admires her. She is truly courageous. She must also be very, very lonely.

Today the only other person in the lobby was a large, very bent-over woman. There was not even anyone at the desk. I was sitting near the door waiting for a friend to take me out, when the bent-over woman came slowly over to me. "What do you do," she asked, "when you don't know what you want to do?"

How do you answer a question like that? I was first surprised. I had given her no answer (for I had none) when my friend drove up. As we drove away, the question haunted me. How the days must drag for many, in spite of the entertainment and planned events. Those things are done by others for you. What can you do from the inside out?

I remember a friend asking why she does not see me often at lunch. "I don't eat much lunch," I replied. "I find three meals a day a bit much for inactive living."

She sighed. "But it breaks the day." I guess that's why food is such an important part of our scheme of things: it breaks the day.

I must not fail to mention one innovation in menu planning. For Mother's Day and Memorial Day, people on one floor were asked to plan the menu. (Cynical me, I think it's easier for food service, since only one choice was given for the day.) The food was the same quality as ever, but wasn't it nice to let the residents have some say-so? We have been good children, thus we can have a part in planning something.

When Will
Our Cry Be Heard?

My daughter has received a lengthy memo stating that the Home has created a new advisory structure composed of six councils, and asking her to serve on a council to meet six times a year. A few excerpts from the memo: "Each council could: appoint task forces assigned a specific planning or problem-solving task, with target dates, for recommendation to the council and to management; recommend to facility administrators future changes in the environment that incorporate the milieu therapy concepts; review the planning process for the hospice feasibility study." My daughter read only the first paragraph of that jargonese. She had attended, by invitation, an early orientation meeting and responded to a questionnaire by saying that the meeting was too long and not very helpful. Orientation meetings have not changed one bit. What good would being on a council do?

The Food Service Committee has already met with the Administrator. They gave him a lot of input concerning the poor quality of dinner meals but got brushed off with vague promises that "it will get better."

The Administrator is inclined to go to committee meetings without being invited and throws a damper over everything. As one person said, "He puts us down so much that we don't feel free to speak out."

The Association is the group to which individuals and committees *can* bring complaints and recommendations, but people feel a damper there, too. The Administrator or Director of Resident Relations attend the meetings, make a few remarks, and ask if anyone has a question. The meeting turns into a regular routine of reading minutes, financial statements, announcements, etc. Nobody ever makes waves.

Why does nobody make waves? I think I know. Since it often takes several months, even a year, to get into some places, many older people feel like doors are shut in their faces. Then, after they enter, they feel as if a door has shut behind. Soon after I came I got off the elevator with three women who live on the other end of the hall. As they turned left and I turned right, I heard one say, vehemently, "I hate this place."

Another spoke in the same tone of voice. "Well, love it. I do. I have no other place to go."

A *listening ear.* We are given one chance to speak in a conference with the Administrator soon after we come. One friend told me that he asked her, "What do you do when you get depressed?" When she said she is rarely depressed, he insisted, "Oh, yes you are. All older people suffer from depression." Again she repeated that she does not get depressed; again he insisted that she must.

"Finally," she told me, "I just said to him that if I feel low, I say my prayers and get busy."

She said she would have said more but was afraid. She comes from another state, and when she first came she was given an undesirable apartment that overlooks the work area where trucks begin deliveries about six in the morning. She objected, and asked for another. The Administrator told her if she didn't like her apartment, she didn't have to stay. There is a long waiting list. She next went to the Director of Resident Relations, who immediately assigned her another apartment.

This woman is a gentle person, unused to discourtesy. After her first conversation with the Administrator regarding the apartment, she has felt trapped and frightened. When someone has been cowed just as she has given up friends and home, she does not recover easily. She is one who fears she will not be allowed to stay.

Mrs. Hinton, not more than seventy-five, talked frankly with me recently. She had heard that this was an unusually desirable place, but she's disappointed because there seems no recourse for improvement. The hush-hush attitude bothers her. She feels it will take a real struggle to bring about improvement. She is on the Food Service Committee. She said, "I have struggled enough in P.T.A., civic affairs, and many other areas trying to help make things better. I'm tired." She also feels trapped, absorbed, her strength slipping from her. "It's so easy to give up, so much easier than to fight." And then, sadly, "But I don't like this state of being. It makes me unhappy."

I urged her not to give up. "It will take time and effort, but we old people must not give up. There are more and more of us and we have the power of the vote," I reminded her. However, that won't solve our problems here, now or in the near future. "Just don't knuckle under," I said. "If nothing can be done by the Food Committee working through the Association and from there to the Administration, then there are enough people to organize on their own and present a petition to a higher level. Such a plan might not work, but we can try. We pay for what we get, after all."

She said as we parted, "You are the best *unloader-oner* I've ever known!" I've never been called that before, but if that has become my role here, so be it.

Many conversations here deal with relations between residents and their children. Several people here have told me about feeling unwanted and put upon by their children. One woman whom I have never seen smile says that her children forget her, that they are glad she is here and out of their way. Another, a younger-older, told me her son took her car and sold it without asking her.

"Was the car in your name?" I asked. She nodded. "Then didn't you have to sign something before it could be sold?" I asked. She nodded again. "Well, you didn't have to sign, did you?"

She sighed, "No, but they felt like I should." Thus, she frets because she does not have a car and blames her children. I am told by long-time residents that complaints about children taking over one's life are common.

My children and I came to an agreement long ago. We enjoy one another, but we enjoy our independence, too. They need have no fear I would live with them. All of them have dogs, and some have cats as well. Too often when I visit, my favorite chair is occupied by a dog. If I spend the night, I don't dare leave my door open or I might find myself with a cozy but unwanted cat for a bedfellow.

I make a wave! Last night I made a wave at Association meeting, though I had no intention of doing so. A suggestion was made by one woman that we have a group blessing for dinner. The president asked for a motion and a second, which were immediately forthcoming. Then she asked if there were any discussion.

I am certainly not against praying, but a scene suddenly flashed through my head: people coming in and being seated, more coming in at intervals, waitresses rushing to write orders and scurrying to bring in early orders, then the bell sounds. A waitress stops in the aisle between tables with a tray full of dishes, the coffee server stops with her pot poised mid-air, another waitress bends over to put dirty dishes in the dishpan on the floor, and a voice says, "We will now have the blessing."

Knowing that many people who did not think having a group blessing was a good idea would still vote for it because they feared somebody might say they were against prayer, I thought a discussion was in order. I raised my hand and went to the mike. "I think a blessing would be impractical in the present situation," I said. "At what point in the dining process would a blessing fit in, with people starting and finishing at different times?" I went on to say that anyone wishing to pray could certainly do so silently, or each table could have their own (as I was sure was already being done).

A vote was called for. It sounded like the no's had it, but since the room is large and some voices not strong, it was decided to have a show of hands as well. The no's definitely had it. When I left the room later, two or three people stopped me to say they were glad I had said what I did. As I continued into the hall, others did the same. Even the President of the Association caught up with me to say how glad she was I had said what I did, that I had said it well and been courageous to do it. I was amazed at her word "courageous." What is courageous about stating your opinion in a democratic society?

Tonight going into dinner, more people spoke to me about my speech. To a special friend I said, "I think it would have been voted down anyway from the way it sounded."

She shook her head. "No, it was very easy to *say* 'no' because you could only be heard by people nearby, but raising your hand could be seen much farther." I concluded that it also must have taken courage for people to do that.

. . . *to prolong independence* . . . This beautiful morning I got up feeling not too poorly. I thought, "It's not so bad being old." I ate breakfast, straightened my apartment, and went down to the lobby to mail some letters. Then I opened my box.

I had a memo from the Administrator. "Starting this month we will begin to have an annual interview between staff and residents whose anniversary date of moving into the Home occurs during that month. The purpose of this interview is to give you the opportunity to communicate your likes and dislikes and to express any problems you may be experiencing. You will be invited to participate, but it is completely optional. In either case, the staff will have an annual review of each resident to determine how to prolong independence."

I noted the words, "in either case." We will be evaluated anyhow. And whatever we say or do, we will not actually be the decision makers about our own futures. I also noted "determine how to prolong independence." In my opinion, the less we have to do with them the better able we will be to prolong our independence!

How do you prolong independence? By straining hands and

arms to carry a heavy tray, by bending over to shove the tray onto the bottom rack of dishes, by tottering on weak knees through the garden? You certainly don't prolong anyone's independence by rebutting every suggestion they make for improvements, by blocking lines of communication between administration and residents and, to a degree, between resident and resident.

Can My Spirit Survive?

Summertime—
When the Living Is
About the Same

Summer has truly come. We will have no more night programs or morning Bible studies until September. A few people are leaving for vacations. One man is going to Sweden, his former home.

The weather got quite warm in early June, and the air conditioning came on—but only for a few days. The maintenance men said the main part had broken down.

"How long will it take to fix it?"

"Don't know. We're working on it."

Meanwhile the weather got hotter and hotter. Some people have colds from sitting too near an electric fan. This morning I heard two women talking as they got their mail. "I'm almost sick from being too hot," said one, "and there aren't enough seats outside."

"Why don't you walk?" suggested the other.

The first shook her head. "You can't walk all day."

Finally, this afternoon, the air conditioning began to function. At dinner the Administrator came into the dining room. "The air conditioning is on," he announced. "Now you can begin to complain about the food."

The usual number of things are going wrong. The large elevator is not working for the second time in two weeks, which means all two hundred of us must use the smaller one to get to dinner. This evening, eight of us from my floor collected in the hall to go down. For several runs, every time the elevator stopped, it was full. Because of my weak knee I sat in one of two chairs by the elevators. Others leaned against the wall. Three more people came from the other end of the hall.

After fifteen minutes of standing, one of the stalwart ones remarked that we could walk down. A few of us said no, *we* couldn't. Just then a woman of ninety-one who is recovering from a recent hip operation came along. She certainly could not walk down seven floors. She was even hesitant about going on the elevator, in case we could not get back up. I gave her my chair.

We waited another five minutes before there was room for us to get on. The elevator was going up, but we got on anyway. We stopped on almost every floor to pick up people, then on the way down stopped again on each floor even though it was already full. The woman with the weak hip held my hand the whole time. She was trembling.

Not only are the elevators not working properly, but the food service is short-staffed for the summer months. Sunday we had about half the number of needed servers. I had to brush crumbs from my chair before I sat down. We waited one hour to be served. By then the kitchen had run out of some of the items we ordered, and the tossed salad had not been drained.

More people are bringing down little brown bags to dinner containing supplementary bits and bites. Some are bringing large bags, perhaps a pie wrapped in foil, even roast beef. More vacancies can be seen—more people are eating out even though they've paid for meals here.

The Food Committee as a group has given up. Mrs. Hinton is totally discouraged. She really has tried to bring about some change but is tired of struggling and feels it is no use. She has been told by some of those who are firmly entrenched here that she is too

outspoken. She told me she has decided to give up fighting and
enjoy life here as well as she can.

In spite of difficulties, some maintain their sense of humor.
The unpalatable, fried, very dry fish continues on the Friday night
menu. Last Friday a small group of us were standing outside the
dining room doors after dinner and one man remarked that he gave
his fish to a cat that wanders about the patio, but even the cat
wouldn't eat it.

The next morning this bit of doggerel, typed on a large index
card, appeared on the bulletin board:

> Who wants a dried-up piece of fish?
> Why every Friday have such a dish?
> When a piece of such fish was given a cat
> She just spat! and spat! and spat!

An artist had illustrated it from the depths of her (or his) soul.
On each corner of the card an ugly cat scowled ferociously, tail
raised as if ready to spring. Two men and two women were seated at
a table. One man was trying to entice a cat to take a piece of fish,
while a determined looking woman was shaking a finger at him and
saying, "No, no, Jack!" The second man was laughing while the
second woman looked bewildered.

Evidently the card was put up late at night or early in the
morning. I went by just as it was taken down by the Administrator
and the President of the Association as they put up some new items.
This effort had a very short life. I wonder if there will be more.

Despair creeps in. Something is happening before my very eyes that
is tearing me apart. Mr. Brown is no longer rebelling, he is suc-
cumbing. He is such a strong character that I never believed this
would happen to him. He is thinking and talking about leaving,
trying another place. I am not urging him one way or the other. I
listen to him and talk things over, try to help him see the odds for
and against each situation. There is some consolation in knowing
you can leave, but he might run into the same problems somewhere
else. Furthermore, he would likely have a long wait getting into

another place. By the time he got in there, this Home might have improved.

The crux of the matter for Mr. Brown is not the poor food or things that interfere with comfort. What eats on him is his loss of freedom and identity. I watch him becoming more and more depressed, giving in to what seems inevitable. He is not easing into the "what's the use?" state without realizing it, like some others. He is very conscious of what is happening to him, knows it is self-destructive, but yet cannot seem to snap back as he did when he first came. For me, watching him succumb is like watching someone with a terminal illness. It breaks my heart. Can I help save him? Can anyone? The only thing I see to do just now is to keep on caring.

The first annual reviews. Six of my women friends have been called for their "anniversary interviews." The Director of Resident Relations is in charge and takes notes. The Administrator was not present at any of the meetings. Also attending were the Chaplain and people from other work areas, although not the same ones every time. Most of these people have had little or no training in working with the elderly. It is a bit much to ask a resident to sit with this group and discuss personal feelings which will be evaluated later by the group or the Director.

A summary of the six conferences I've heard about goes like this:

The interviewing group is seated in the conference room and seem a little ill at ease when you take your seat. The Director makes a few remarks and then asks if there is anything you would like to say about yourself and your life here. The idea is to *discuss* your feelings.

Mrs. A. told them she did not like the evening meal but soft-pedalled everything else.

Mrs. B., who has been here five years, told them plainly that almost everything is unsatisfactory these days. They listened without comment.

Mrs. C., who came for a year and has now gone, stated her complaints with vigor.

Mrs. D. made two visits. The first time she went, only the Chaplain and two kitchen supervisors were present. These supervisors attend to serving food and do some cooking. They also are supposed to oversee the dining room and waitresses but are not in the dining room often. Mrs. D. sat down and they waited a bit. The Chaplain finally said the Director could not be present, and so Mrs. D. left.

A second appointment was made. This time the Director was present, also those who were there the first time. Mrs. D. stated that she is not entirely unhappy here, because she does not allow herself to be, but she does not feel at home here even though this is supposed to be as near like home as possible. She is a native of the city; some of her family are here. She has been a principal in the school system. One of the major things she deplores is the authoritarian atmosphere. She spoke plainly.

Mrs. E. is a native of this city, several years a resident of the Home, a younger-older, quite alert in every way, very fair minded, generous, and considerate. She feels this is truly her home but she finds many things have gone wrong unnecessarily and there is great need for improvement. She frankly expressed her views. She is one of the few who will speak out. If we ever come to the stage where we feel we can organize and approach the proper authorities, she will participate, I hope.

Mrs. F. and I were discussing the conferences before she was called for hers. She is from another state, and only came to this home because she has a daughter in this city. She came about the same time I did. She is very disappointed and finds the Home much overrated. Of course, her daughter could only judge by what she could see or read about it, which is truly deceptive. You don't see the flaws until you live here a while. Mrs. F. has kept most of her distress to herself, for she wants to be near her daughter and does not want her daughter worrying about her.

She is quite capable of making a fair judgment. Her husband taught in a well-known university, and she has done specialized work in many libraries, including the Library of Congress. Here she has had a lot of trouble with her bathroom ventilator, and an odor from her heating unit has never been remedied. She said she wanted to be honest in the interview, but since she has been in the hospital lately with a heart condition, she felt too weak to buck the establishment. I told her she didn't even have to go to the interview if she didn't feel like it.

"Oh, but I feel I ought to go," she said. Others have said the same. The memo said that participation is entirely voluntary, but the feeling is that we will get "demerits" or somehow be discriminated against if we do not go.

She went, and managed to let them know some of the things she objects to, including the problems with her heating unit. She got the usual response, "Maintenance is working on it." They have never come to her room, and so we wonder exactly where they are working.

(One of the maintenance workers told me he could do nothing about my bathroom ventilator not working because the fan on the roof that draws the air out is no good and there will be no money for a new one until next April. If the trouble is on the roof, does that mean that the ventilators for twelve floors are not working? Now I wonder if our air is polluted.)

Mrs. F. has become depressed since her interview. Though she had a heart condition before she came, I feel it has worsened because of the situation here. She sees no hope of improvement. I can see her weakening, going downhill. Sometimes for several days at a time she doesn't come down for meals. The fear of being sent to the next level of care has her in its grip. I tell her that that is not the only place she could go, there are better. Nevertheless, she fears a sudden heart attack will trap her.

A *departure.* The man who joked about feeding his fish to the cat left us. He and his wife moved to another home in a different state. He has been in bad health for some time, although he can still go on his own, and his mental processes are not in the least impaired. Both he and his wife are intelligent and delightful company. They had many friends here.

Not long ago, however, his wife had a bad flare-up of arthritis in one knee and had to be in the hospital for a while. When she came back here, she was restricted in the amount of walking she could do, so only went to the dining room for dinner, depending on the use of a walking stick.

While his wife was slowly improving, the husband had a virus and, in order to avoid any undue strain for his wife, he went to the nursing center on the grounds here. In a few days he recovered, was able to be up, and needed no special attention. His doctor dismissed him. He called here to report he was ready to return. The Assistant Administrator told him he could not. When asked why, she gave no good reason, only saying that she had the final say so. The man was kept at the nursing center three more days, up and dressed and needing no attention at all, with nothing to do. It cost him $50.00 per day in addition to rent on his apartment here. There was no reason why he should have been prevented from returning. He should have come on anyway. Such unfair authority should be defied. But when one is old and ill, one yields.

The wife's knee did not improve as they had hoped and the doctor said she might come to need a wheelchair. If they remained here, she would have to go to the intermediary level of care in the building next to this one and share a double room with another woman, while her husband remained here. They elected to go to a retirement home where people can have a wheelchair if they can operate it on their own.

What happened to these wonderful people is a good example of how a human being's sense of security and well being goes downhill.

A *week of petty annoyances*. One elevator was out for thirty minutes last Sunday, making some late for church. Wednesday all the current went off again, and both elevators were out for an hour. Eva Dean confided that since she came she has not been able to take a shower, because the cold tap in her shower doesn't work. Apparently valves need to be replaced. Somebody is "working on it."

The air conditioner continues to function erratically. One day the temperature was above ninety and we were pleasantly cool. Today a cool front came through and we froze.

The dining room is still short of staff. Last night our waitress whisked our plates from under our noses before we finished our main course, then wiped our tables with a dirty gray cloth as we ate our desserts.

Mr. Brown asked today about a second key to his unit; he originally asked for it four months ago. It has not yet been made. I tell myself that there are other places much worse—but it's like an earache. Knowing somebody else has a worse one doesn't lessen your own discomfort.

Safety *Last*

One woman told me recently that in spite of all the problems here, she stays because she feels so safe. Is she? Are any of us? At least three-fourths of the first floor walls are glass. The area is well-lit, but that did not keep thieves from stealing seven batteries from cars in our parking area one night. Inside, I doubt that burglars would find much worth taking, but other physical aspects of the Home are not what I'd call "safe."

As I said before, we have only two elevators for two hundred people, and one or the other is often out of service. The elevators are also used to haul laundry carts, big vacuum cleaners, and garbage cans. One day last week Mr. Brown and two other men were waiting for an elevator. As it opened, a janitor pushed out a big vacuum cleaner, almost hitting one of the men. He jumped back quickly and fell flat on the floor. Mr. Brown took him to the doctor to be checked. Fortunately no bones were broken.

One day I got on the small elevator which was already carrying a large laundry cart. Since it reached from the front of the elevator to the back, I had to squeeze by it to get in and had barely enough room to stand. When the maid pushed it off two floors later, it moved against me. "Look out!" I exclaimed involuntarily.

"Lady," she answered crossly, "I can't tell which way the wheels are going when I push it." How safe is that?

Falls—and failures. Within the past week two crises have occurred that cannot be overlooked.

On Monday night Mrs. Saunders did not come to dinner. The other three women at her table thought nothing of that. People miss one night quite often. Therefore, since none of them live on her floor, no one went by to check on her.

Outside each apartment is a small device about one inch by one-and-a-half inches, called the "stat check." Half red and half white, it remains on the red position at all times except when residents move it to white each morning to show they are able to change it. The floor leader (a resident) checks each door about 9 A.M. and slides the stat back to red. If any stat has not been moved, the floor leader reports to the lobby desk.

Tuesday morning Mrs. Saunders' floor leader found her stat check on red. She immediately notified the receptionist, who went to the office of the Director of Resident Relations. She was out, but the receptionist told her secretary to put in a call for a nurse from the nursing center on the grounds. She *forgot*. The receptionist did not go upstairs, either, to unlock Mrs. Saunders' door and check on her.

Finally, Tuesday evening when she failed to show up for dinner, her tablemates decided to check on her themselves. One of them called her son, who lives nearby. Having heard nothing from his mother and getting no answer from her phone, he called the Home. The receptionist discovered that the secretary had never called a nurse and did so himself. The son and nurse arrived at about the same time, and the receptionist went with them to her room.

Mrs. Saunders was found lying on the floor by the bed where she had fallen, in a semi-conscious condition. As well as she could recall, she had fallen the night before. She must have been there twenty-four or more hours before she was found. She was taken to the hospital and is doing fine, but this has disturbed all of us greatly.

Even the Administrator is perturbed. By the time Mrs. Saunders went to the hospital, all the staff except the receptionist had left for the day. The Administrator asked the floor leader the next day for her version of what had happened, and she asked if he wanted her to attend the staff meeting he had called about it. "No," he replied. "I don't want you to hear the language I'm going to use."

Our second crisis involved Mrs. Lacy, who thinks she had some kind of fall or seizure. She fell in her room and a maid cleaning next door heard her and called the desk. A volunteer was on duty. He came up, and he and the maid put Mrs. Lacy on her bed. She insisted that the volunteer not notify the office, that she felt all right. He should have notified the office anyway but yielded to her request.

When I went down in the elevator that night, Mrs. Lacy was telling the other passengers about her fall. She ate dinner as usual, and then on the elevator going back to her room she became very weak. She had to ask someone to walk her to her room. That woman said later that the reason Mrs. Lacy won't let anyone report her fall and also the reason she made the effort to go down to dinner is that she fears she will be taken to the nursing home.

The second crisis was not as serious as the first—Mrs. Lacy is apparently fine now. I link them together, however, because both times the person on call made a serious error which could have been life-threatening. We have volunteer receptionists often. This would be fine if they were well trained, keenly aware, and capable of acting according to instructions. Since they are not, we are particularly vulnerable when they are on duty.

Volunteers are the only persons on duty at night. A volunteer comes to the receptionist desk about 5 P.M. and remains until nine, when another volunteer comes on emergency duty until seven the next morning. We have no patrol or security guard at night. The night volunteer, often a woman, stays in a room behind the desk where there is a television and a cot where she can sleep.

Volunteers are also on duty every weekend, for no staff members—even maintenance personnel—are here. I have often wondered what would happen if a bad leak should occur, the heat or air conditioning go off, or an elevator quit working. These things happen only too frequently, but dangers to our health are even greater on these days. The weekend that Mrs. Roberts broke her hip last spring, only a volunteer was here to help. He seemed not to know that a person who has fallen should not be moved until a nurse or medic has examined her. He picked Mrs. Roberts up and put her in a chair, then again into a wheelchair before professional help arrived. Volunteers should be better informed.

Know a good plumber? This afternoon I went to the far end of the hall to visit a friend before dinner. She was very pale, and her voice sounded weak. When the time came to go, she could not get up from the sofa where she sat. She kept trying but could not make it. I soon realized she was ill. I could not help her up, because my own arms are so weak I do well to get *myself* out of a chair. She did not want me to even try—likely we would have both landed on the floor.

I brought her a washcloth for her face and asked her to let me call the desk for help, or her daughter, but she insisted that I just go to dinner and leave her. I said I would eat, then come back to check on her. On my way down, I called her daughter. She said she was just getting ready to call her mother anyway and would not say I had called. When I went by later, her daughter was there and had called a doctor. An ambulance was on its way to take her mother to the hospital.

It turns out my friend has a staph infection which is not serious and can be easily treated. Where did she get it? Who knows?

I do know that when I went to wet her a cloth for her face, I noticed that four or more square feet of plaster in the wall behind her toilet is torn out, exposing the pipes inside. I asked about it, and my friend said they are working on a leak in the drain. I asked how long they have had the wall out, and she said three weeks.

Could there be staph inside that space?

In my own shower, the drain in the floor does not operate

correctly. More often than not, all the water does not drain away.
Instead it stands there, a dirty color, and occasionally overflows.
Then I call maintenance and they come with a plunger to squoosh
it out. The water has to go down about seventy feet, but I don't know
if the people beneath me also have trouble. I don't like to ask people
I don't know very well about their bathroom drains!

I'd like to know just how much bacteria lurks around here
and there amid worn-out plumbing. Actually, I'd rather not.

Moving into Autumn

August is gone. For three weeks I had a wonderful visit with my daughter in another state. Now, on my return, many people say they missed me and are glad to have me back. I missed them, too. I truly like and love many of the people here. I do not, however, say I am glad to be "home," as many say when they return. I cannot call it home.

My first night back we watched a television program in the music room, on which a panel discussed the popular subject of "Aging." The panel consisted of a professor of sociology at a local university, the director of a number of retirement homes (including the one in which I live), and a Ph.D. student in the field of gerontology. What they had to say was good, but only up to a point. Those of us who watched the program agreed: *they know so little about us and how we feel about it all.*

Visiting "outside" has made me conscious again of how little contact most people, especially children, have with older people. I believe children should associate with the aged from infancy, whenever possible. They respond well to older people if the situation is favorable for response.

Yesterday, for example, I was visiting the playground of a nearby kindergarten. Sometimes I pick up my walking stick in such a way that the curved handle is turned forward instead of backwards, and I just leave it that way. In the park, a little boy of about four came over to me and said, "Hi, old lady."

"Hi, yourself," I answered.

He reached for my stick, turned it around, and handed it back to me. As he did so, he said "You are carrying that stick the wrong way." I thanked him, and we went our separate ways. In our encounter we could both have been eighty—or four. We had communicated in the right way.

Mr. Brown likes children, and soon after he got here he was asked by his church to permit a group of eight children to visit him in his apartment one Sunday morning. He was quite willing, although he had not finished unpacking. The children came and sat on cartons, chairs, and even on his bed. They chatted with him for about fifteen minutes and gave him some paper flowers they had made. He still has them. That sort of thing provides so much more contact between generations than when groups come in to sing for us and then leave.

Children need to know older people, and older people need to know children. On my floor there happen to be two great-grandmothers of the same two-and-a-half-year-old child. Whenever she comes to visit, she scampers from one apartment to the other, entertaining the rest of us on her way. Other young children come to visit on our floor, too, of course, but are usually kept inside the apartments. When this child comes, we all enjoy her visits.

It occurs to me that a fascinating learning experience called Simulation could help younger people understand how older people feel, by putting themselves in older people's shoes. Such things as being blindfolded or wearing gauze to blur vision, wearing earplugs, wrapping knees with elastic bandages to make them stiff and difficult to bend, wearing plastic gloves to inhibit touch—all these would let people experience some of the awkward parts of aging. Of course simulation experiences afford only the difficulty of movement, not the chronic pain and stiffness than accompany these handicaps. It would be a start toward understanding, however.

Our conference on aging. A big two-day conference on aging was held here last week. A few residents served as hostesses, but none of us was invited to attend. Delegates were housed elsewhere, but workshops met here and in the other three buildings of our complex. Luncheon was served in our dining room, and so we had to be out by noon. Then the visitors came at one and partook of an elegant smorgasbord. Five outside people came in to prepare food, and the price was very low—they probably used the chicken that was intended for the residents' next dumpling dinner! After the guests left, we were invited to come in and eat leftover sandwiches.

The kitchen was painted before the conference and dried just in time. When the door swings open, we get a glimpse of the far wall. Very nice.

On the Friday before the conference, it was announced that the carpet in the lobby, near the elevators, and in the gallery would be shampooed Saturday night. All outside doors would be locked at 9 P.M. and no one could get back inside after that. The Administrator remarked that anyone left out could take a bedroll to sleep in. Mr. Brown whispered that he was tempted to stay out until eleven, and if they refused to let him back in, go to an expensive hotel and send them the bill. I was sorry he didn't.

Now that the conference is over, things are back to normal. By that I mean, not especially comfortable. A late September cold front came through just before the conference began; therefore, the heat was turned on. After the visitors left Tuesday afternoon, it was turned off—even though it was cool enough every morning for a week to need heat. One woman from my floor went down to see the head of maintenance. She said she did not understand why the heat was on for visitors and off for residents.

"I take that as a personal insult," he growled.

"I didn't mean it as an insult," she replied. "It's just a fact.

There was heat for the visitors, and now there's none for residents."

He mumbled a bit and said he'd have to take it up with the Administrator. We stayed cold until the weather changed.

Another fall. It was about time for it to happen. It's to be expected ever so often. At dinner last night I was surprised when a new woman suddenly fell right by my chair. She had been sitting directly behind me, therefore I did not see if she just fell from her chair or had gotten up to leave when she fell. She did not seem to be hurt and started to get up. She is very heavy and was having difficulty in rising, and so Mr. Brown went to ask the volunteer on duty to help. Everyone else pretended nothing had happened.

It is quite a long walk from the dining room to the lobby, and there is no intercom in the dining room—although most falls occur there. A person who had a heart attack could easily die before someone could bring help from the desk. (Most of us here, after all, are not fast walkers.)

When Mr. Brown asked the man at the desk for a wheelchair and assistance, the man hesitated to leave the desk. He asked Mr. Brown to take the wheelchair back with him. Mr. Brown informed him that residents are not allowed to do that. The volunteer did not know about that rule.

They brought a chair back, helped the woman in, and in a few minutes she walked out of the dining room alone. She was more embarrassed than hurt. Several of us remained behind to discuss the incident. It worries us that to get a wheelchair through the dining room in case of emergency means moving several tables, chairs, and even dishpans, which takes time that could mean the difference between life and death. It worries us that there is no intercom. It worries us most of all that if there *is* a procedure for handling dining room emergencies, the volunteers have not been informed.

I don't want to appear curious . . . This morning two women on the elevator with me were discussing last night's fall. As we reached the ground floor one said to me, "You were sitting near where she fell, weren't you? Was she hurt?"

I said the woman had not seemed to be hurt, and we discussed it a little more. Then the woman who had asked about it said, "I didn't mean to be curious, I just wanted to know if she was hurt."

Her remark threw light on something that Mr. Brown and I have often discussed: the fact that whenever *anything* like that happens here, people seem to pretend nothing has happened and have little to say about it afterwards. Is it because they don't want to appear curious? Or because they don't want to be involved?

I said to the woman, "We are born with curiosity. You have a right to be curious; you should know about things that happen here."

After I got my mail, I went upstairs and rested. I am weary. Weary of trying to sort things out. Weary of searching for reasons and causes. Weary of seeking solutions. And, I think, most of all weary of thinking.

Humorous interludes. Mr. Brown received the following memo for men only from the Director of Resident Relations, who is working on a graduate degree:

> I am writing a research paper on the effects of retirement on older males. I have five questions I would like to ask you and would like to do so in a group setting. I am asking ten men at a time to meet me in the conference room to discuss the subject. I hope you will be free to come and discuss the questions below with me on October 29 at 10 A.M.

There were five questions, among them "What were your feelings the first morning you did not have a job to go to?" "What is the worst thing about not having a job?" and "What is the best thing about not having a job?" A few men went to the first meeting and the Director did not appear. She had forgotten all about it.

This place smacks strongly of being a research center in gerontology. If we are to live in a laboratory rather than in a Home, we should be so informed when we apply. Mr. Brown and his friends ignored the questionnaire entirely. But we had fun coming up with outlandish answers he *could* have given to the questions.

A second bit of doggerel appeared on the bulletin board last week, printed on a plain index card and unsigned. It read:

> This old man is going to die,
> All from eating hamburger pie.
> Whatever was in it
> 'Twas sin to put in it,
> So now we are going to cry.

A funny cartoon at the top showed a round ring for a table with a biscuit on a plate. The heads and shoulders of an unhappy man and woman stared at it. Above his head was an exclamation point and above hers, a question mark.

Evidently the card was put on the bulletin board the night before, for Mr. Brown saw it when he went down to breakfast and told me about it. He said few people who saw it said anything about it. I saw it when I went down for the mail about ten. No one else was around. By lunchtime it had been taken down.

The next morning, a third verse was put up before breakfast.

> Did you ever have dumplings without any chicken?
> If so, you'd better look in the kitchen.
> They will bring you some chicken if you ask them to,
> Something you ought not to have to do.
> It's all very bewitchin'.

This one showed an old, bald, thin-faced man with a look of bewilderment on his face and a woman with lots of curly hair, a plump face, and a double chin resting on her cupped hands propped by her elbows. She wore a frown.

That card, too, was down by lunchtime. That night, however, as we waited in the gallery for the doors to open for dinner, a man near me remarked on it. People are beginning to take notice.

A magazine cartoon is on the bulletin board now. It shows a man running for dear life and two women trying to catch him, calling wildly, "Wait!" It is in no way critical of the institution and has nothing to do with food. It has stayed on the board nearly a week.

The food again. I have promised myself several times not to write about the food service again, but this time I cannot refrain. We have ice cream or sherbet about three times a week—a very good brand. Several hours before a meal is served, it is placed in small aluminum dishes with a stem, then put back into the freezer. Although brought to our tables long before we finish our meal, the ice cream is usually still hard when we begin to eat it.

Last night a waitress brought in a tray of fifteen servings and set it on a vacant table while she cleared some dishes. The tray was unbalanced and fell to the floor. A few dishes fell upright, but most fell onto the carpet upside down or rolled under another table. The waitress picked them back up and put them on the tray. Then she went across the dining room to tables that had not seen them fall and proceeded to serve them! Those of us who did see it agreed not to tell the people who ate it. We wouldn't want to know. Why is no one responsible to oversee this dining room? There ought to be a law—and probably there is.

Democracy for the elderly. Now our Administrator has assumed the power of veto. For several years the Home has received twelve free tickets to each of a variety of concerts in a large theatre here. The tickets are worth two hundred dollars for the season. Those who used the tickets paid a dollar each and were taken to the entertainment in a bus belonging to the Home.

Last month the person in charge of this deal was notified that complimentary tickets are no longer available, but the tickets could be purchased for two hundred dollars. After conversations here and there, the Administrator offered to lend the money to the Association out of a fund he has, to be paid back in small amounts over a long period of time. Since the Association only meets every other month, the executive committee asked each floor to have a meeting to discuss his offer.

The meetings were held, and a majority voted *on each floor* not to accept his offer. The reason given in every case was that we did not deem it fair for the Association to pay for the entertainment of the few. Let the few who wanted to go to the entertainments buy their own tickets. It was felt that a loan would only be acceptable if it would benefit all.

Now we have been informed that the Administrator has "vetoed" the report of the executive committee and is going to loan the Association the money anyway. Most of us can't accept his power of veto on any grounds. Why take the time of the executive committee and waste all that time in meetings?

My Spirit is heavy. Last spring I was in the hospital briefly. While there, one of my doctors asked how I like the Home, and I answered frankly. He seemed glad to have my reactions and said that people who work with the elderly still have much to learn. I told him that I often jotted down thoughts or incidents about the Home. He said, "That's a good idea. Keep it up. I will be interested in reading what you write. After all, who can tell what it is like to live there better than an old person?"

Without even thinking, I said, "I may have to do it just to save myself." At that time I had no idea what I was trying to save myself from. Now I know. With only a few years left, perhaps only months or even days, my time is pure gold. No matter how long or short the time, there is not enough of it to do all the reading I want to do, all the visiting with other people on a one-to-one basis as well as in groups. I rebel against being restricted by programs and activities, resent being under stress from my environment. Tonight I come face to face with my aloneness here and I have to ask myself: can I survive?

Final Act

Transitions

A number of people have left in the last few weeks because they were not satisfied here and desired a better home.

Eva Dean, my best friend who sat at our dinner table, left today. We will miss her. She was one of the most stimulating persons I've ever known. Even her last day here had an unpleasant incident. She went down to do a final laundry, and the floor of the laundry was covered in water. She asked a janitor in the hall to mop it up, and he said he would get a mop, but she'd have to mop it herself. She told him that indeed she would not mop, so he grumpily did it.

As she left, she stopped by to speak with the Director of Resident Relations out of concern for whoever may get her unit next. At no time since she came has she been able to get cold water from the tap in her shower. She reported it many times, without result. Finally she bought a small tub and put it on the floor of the shower stall. To bathe, she mixed cold water from the lavatory with hot from the shower and managed, with the use of a pitcher, to rinse off. Somewhat primitive, something like a bucket hanging from a tree

in the jungle, only her water had to be lifted up by hand. She mentioned it on leaving because she feared that a new person, not knowing she could not get cold water, might get scalded. The Director
promised to have it attended to, and when a new person moves in,
I shall ask about it.

The Nelsons have also gone. He was one of Mr. Brown's
particular friends. I spoke to him a few days before they left and said
that although I was sorry to see them go, I hoped they would be
better situated in the new place. He had an operation last year to
remove his larynx, and now he speaks through his esophagus. Sadly
he said, "And I thought I would be here the rest of my life." I felt a
wave of compassion for him. He is so thin. His days are not only
numbered because of his age but because of his physical condition.
I doubt if I will ever see him again.

Their last day, too, had its difficulties. A week before they
left, the Nelsons made the usual arrangements with the office concerning the day and hour they planned to move. They were moving
in the late morning. For some reason, a man resident who is usually
very helpful when people move took over the big elevator and operated it all morning. He would not let the Nelsons' movers use it,
saying that people had to go up and down for lunch, thus the movers
had to wait. Naturally, the bill ran up for overtime, more than a
hundred dollars. The office was at fault for scheduling a move near
lunchtime, and the man for assuming undue authority. The Nelsons had to pay, however. The Nelsons said they were going to
ask the Administrator to pay the overtime, but I doubt that he
will pay it.

They were so tired when they finally got away. Mr. Brown
was with them as they waited to go. They stopped by the office to
say goodbye to the Administrator and Mrs. Nelson remarked po-
litely, "We are sorry to go."

"No you're not," the Administrator replied. "If you were, you
wouldn't go."

Another wedding. Mr. Judson's courting paid off. He is the man who
went to Mrs. Parks' apartment and had to wait in the hall while she

put on her shoes. After a short time they were engaged and announced they would be married soon. Since then it has been on
again, off again as far as a wedding date was concerned. Both have
family here, and after a conference or two with them, the couple
announced they would wait a while to marry. Before long he gave
her a ring, which she proudly showed.

Each had an efficiency apartment on separate floors. A few
weeks ago an apartment with a living room became available on our
floor and was assigned to them. It was redecorated, and they moved
in. Between them they had enough furniture to make it quite
attractive.

Early last week they announced the wedding would occur
Sunday, after morning worship, in the parlor of the church they
attend. Only relatives were invited. A champagne breakfast would
follow in a hotel, and they would remain in the hotel for a two-day
honeymoon. Then, late Friday afternoon, the bride became ill. She
had overworked getting the apartment ready. (She is eighty-four, he
is eighty-two.) He was seen carrying a supper tray up to her. Saturday nobody saw or heard from either of them. Sunday morning
dawned bright and beautiful, an ideal wedding day, but we got no
news. At Sunday dinner, how tongues wagged! Had the wedding
come off? Would it be postponed? No one had seen them.

Monday it was rumored that the wedding had come off as
planned, and that Mr. and Mrs. Judson would return to the home
Tuesday. But they were not seen in the dining room Tuesday or
Wednesday. By this time the main speculation was where they
would sit together in the dining room, for they had sat at different
tables before. Would someone at a table where one of them had sat
leave so they could sit together, or would they get places at another
table altogether? Also, if Mr. Judson left his old table, would a man
or woman get his place—and if a woman, which woman? In spite
of our having so few men, three men and one woman were at his
old table.

Tonight, Thursday, six people from our floor arrived at the
elevators about the same time to go down to dinner. An up elevator
stopped, and we all got on to ride up to be sure of places going
down. As we stopped at our floor again going down, there stood Mr.

Judson at the back of a wheelchair, with the bride sitting in it—pretty as a picture and beaming. There was no room on the elevator for them, and we passed them by.

We learned later that the bride has phlebitis and must not walk for a while. This morning at breakfast, Mr. Brown heard two women talking at the next table. They apparently had reported the wheelchair to the Administrator, who seemed not to know about it. They said his response was, "Did they do that?" Nothing more. Mr. Brown and I think she should be allowed to use it, and we hope she will soon recover so they can stroll into the dining room arm in arm or holding hands, whichever they prefer. All the world loves a lover.

Anniversaries

My year is up. When I started writing, I thought I should allow a year to observe things fairly. I wish I could say things are better, but the overall picture has not improved. I have decided to leave eventually, as soon as I can find another place—a smaller one in a smaller town, without a long waiting list—but first I want to help Mr. Brown find himself a place. Many are leaving—those who can find another place. People who have been here for many years say it is definitely going downhill, and most agree the place needs a thorough inspection from top to bottom.

Would an inspection really reveal the problems?

This Home reminds me of a beautiful peach with a rose-colored peeling. The grounds outside are lovely, the facility is pleasing to the eye—especially at night with lights on outside and in. When a woman from a distant city came with my daughter to bring me home one evening, she almost gasped, "What a gorgeous place!"

You have to bite into the peach to find out there's a worm inside.

Happy anniversary to the Home. The fifteenth anniversary of the opening of the Home is upon us. People who regularly act as hosts and hostesses are busy recruiting others to greet visitors to various functions, but since we are asked to volunteer for an hour at a time, many decline. Few can stand that long.

We will have three major functions: a dinner on Wednesday night with special invited guests such as trustees and their spouses or other important people connected with the operation of the Home, an open house on Thursday for friends of residents and interested persons, and a tea on Sunday afternoon to climax the festivities, for any who want to come. Vespers will follow on Sunday evening.

At the Association meeting last night, the head of the Hospitality Committee asked residents to make cookies for the open house and tea. Immediately someone pointed out that very few of us have ovens in which to bake—only those with full apartments. Then she suggested that those who do have ovens could bake for those who don't. Someone else pointed out that since few of us bake, very few of us have baking pans. There is also the problem of shopping for ingredients. She dismissed that with, "Well, you can work it out."

Indignation was high on all floors following the meeting. Our floor leader said she would not even ask us to consider making cookies. One floor wrote a letter to the Hospitality Committee suggesting that cookies be baked by one of the cooks in the kitchen whose cookies are quite good and that they be paid for by food service. We shall see what happens.

Anniversary, part two. Many of the women, including the President of the Association, have pretty clothes. Those with evening dresses welcome an opportunity to wear them. We, thus, were not surprised when the President of the Association told floor leaders to ask all women who would to wear evening dresses to the Anniversary Dinner. Those on our floor did not want to wear evening dresses even if

we had them, nor did many others, but here and there at the dinner
I spotted a pretty long dress, and all at the head table wore them.

The tables were attractively decorated, and the girls serving
wore hair nets and fresh, mended uniforms. They were courteous
and even, insofar as they were able to be, efficient. The food was
good, with chicken the main dish. (Nobody expected prime rib.)

Speeches gave the history of the Home and told of its many
accomplishments. Slides were shown of the grounds, the building,
and of smiling people in various settings. (Mr. Tucker on our floor
was one of the smiling faces. He confided to Mr. Brown that he did
not want to be, but his daughter said he should. He also said she
has persuaded him to leave a good bit in his will to the Home, which
he does not want to do.)

For dessert we had a beautiful cake. The woman who has
been here the longest cut it, then the waitresses passed it around. In
a lull in the conversation a voice piped up, "I want my cake. I want
my cake."

It was Mrs. Tucker, who was so upset the night of the storm.
She is so very deaf that she doesn't know how loud she talks. She is
also not easily pacified and wants what she wants when she wants it.
Since she never engages in conversation, it is difficult to judge how
much she reasons, but she certainly does where food is concerned.
She always appears in the gallery about thirty minutes before each
meal and eats well.

As she continued her litany, our Director of Resident Relations got up and went to her. Kneeling beside her, she patted Mrs.
Tucker gently but to no avail. Finally the Director caught a passing
waitress by the smock and got a piece of cake. Mrs. Tucker ate
it with her usual relish, got up abruptly in the middle of things,
and left.

Otherwise all went well. Afterwards, many of us spoke to the
people at the head table and residents who helped make the evening
a success. Compliments flowed freely like sparkling wine. Then we
went slowly to our rooms, chatting on the way and lingering in the
halls. It was indeed an entertaining, pleasant evening.

The next day we had Open House most of the day. Our special guests were people invited from other homes in the vicinity. Only punch and cookies were served, and since few people came there were enough (even though none of us had made any). We were asked to leave our apartment doors open so guests could see them if they wished. Residents with friends in these other homes and those with unusually lovely apartments and fine furniture did so. The rest of us went about business as usual.

From the remarks of some visitors, they felt we were rather showing off. Other homes are plainer and do not have the outside surroundings to compare with ours. As I have said before, our place does give an outsider the impression of luxury, style, and perhaps even a touch of wealth. They should have stayed for dinner!

Today, Sunday, the final event of the Anniversary Celebration was held, a tea from three to five to which all friends of the Home were invited. Many people came, so that the lobby, hall, and a small room near the elevators were jammed. The receiving line was in the small room. Extra chairs had been placed against the walls in the lobby, and the usual hard seats were in the gallery. Most people stood anyway.

A long table for refreshments was set up in the hall near the elevators. As I left the elevator I was goggle-eyed at what I beheld: a beautiful silver punch bowl on a lace cloth, surrounded by artistic flower arrangements and plates of goodies. My first impression was "My, I did not know the Home owned such as this." Eventually I learned that all the finery had been rented.

The catered food was delicious, especially the dainty sandwiches. Mr. Brown and I came down with several others from our floor, and we really enjoyed it. I fear we were even greedy. We don't have dinner Sunday nights, so we thought we'd just make it our supper. We stood by the table when not many were around and ate a bit, and then wandered to chat with groups here and there, coming back to eat more later. (One man who is considered peculiar actually filled his coat pockets with little sandwiches and even sticky sweets.) Not only was it delightful to enjoy such delicacies for a change, but I think we felt a sort of vengeance, as if we were getting even with the food people.

Perhaps we were thinking, too, that tomorrow night we'll have canned spinach with thick chicken dumplings, and the green water from the undrained spinach will mix in with the gravy of the dumplings. We have gotten a lot of enjoyment from the Anniversary Celebration. We must now be thankful for our daily bread—even if at times it is a bit green.

Goodbye to a Friend

If Mr. Brown doesn't get away soon, I fear he will either challenge the Administrator to a duel or have a stroke of apoplexy. For a while I was afraid he would break. He became very depressed. Now that he has made up his mind to leave, he has rallied his forces. He looked at a number of places nearby and some not so near before he chose an apartment about a mile away. He did not want to get into another undesirable place.

We hate to separate, but I have definitely decided to go, too. Knowing we can leave helps a lot. We can brace ourselves to put up with what we have to for a while longer. Even the food.

Mr. Brown's emotional state, however, has become much less stable. Until about two months ago, he could snap out of depression quickly. Now he is frequently in a state of gloom. He does not laugh as much, and when we are together he lapses into short periods of silence. Now that he has found a place to go that suits him, he has taken on some new life, but he is not the way he used to be. Packing his belongings is a burden for him. He frets over what to keep and what not to keep. He cannot keep at packing for very long, and his movements are much slower than two months ago.

My windows face the entrance of the building, and I can see the parking area. Sometimes I recognize Mr. Brown below. He has trouble with his knees and walks slowly and carefully, like a very old man. I know that his mind is ahead of his body. I know how hard it is for him to accept. I know he is rebelling too strongly. But I cannot help him. I turn away and occupy my mind with other things.

Although he is only moving a mile, he is packing as if he were going to China. Each small box is tied with rope and labeled, and he has many boxes. Even with plenty of time on his hands, that isn't necessary.

His nervousness and weariness are beginning to get on my nerves, though I hate to admit it. I find myself getting edgy, having trouble being patient. He comes to my apartment more often, though he does not stay as long, and he goes over and over what he should take and what he should discard. He also talks of the past— of how much better it would be if such and such had not happened, of what he and his wife could be doing now if she had not died "so young." (She was in her early sixties, but that seems young when you are eighty.)

Often during the day if I feel unusually tired or if my arthritis is bothering me, I will lie down. When Mr. Brown comes he knocks softly three times, and if I don't answer he knocks again three times. If I still do not answer, he goes away. Up to now there have been few times when I have not answered. Now I find myself dreading his knock. I think, "I can't take it, I just can't." Then, ashamed of myself, I say, "It won't be long. Surely I can hold out for a few more weeks." More and more, however, I turn a deaf ear. I feel guilty, however, that I've done so.

Why haven't I enough inner resources to combat this? Is not my friendship able to bear his burdens? I seem to be able to share the burdens of some others and still maintain my balance. But with Mr. Brown, I care so much that his pain exhausts me.

I would not for anything let him know that he is a trial to me. Often when he gets up to go he says, "I mustn't worry you with my troubles." I try to comfort him by saying that he doesn't bother me, but I believe he senses that he does. He cannot seem to help himself.

What a relief it will be not to hear that soft knock on my door—and how sad I will be not to hear it. At times I am a burden to myself. I wish I could let go and cry as a child cries.

I have never seen anyone here cry, though I am sure some do. As we get older, we cry less (unless we are senile). We learn better and better how to inhibit our feelings, show self-control, how not to weep. Judging by my own feelings, however, I feel that I often do cry, inside. That makes it much harder. My tears are dry.

Tears that are not shed go away slowly and return frequently. Such suffering I cannot adequately describe. I imagine that many old people in this world cry dry tears much of the time.

That is how I weep for Mr. Brown. I cry dry tears for him.

A time of worry. Mr. Brown moved out a month ago, and I am almost ready to leave, too. I will spend next month with my out-of-state daughter, then move into a Home near the coast. Will it be better? I shall see. . . .

Meanwhile, I am worried about Mr. Brown. Last Sunday he drove down to a nearby town to have dinner with his sister-in-law. She is an excellent cook and fixes delightful Sunday midday meals. He called me that night and said he had indigestion. He supposed he had overeaten. Last night (Monday), he called and said that he was still not feeling well and that he was eating very little. I asked if he needed anything and he said he thought he would feel well enough today to go shopping. This afternoon he called to say he still felt bad and would like for his niece and me to get a few things for him and bring them over this evening.

When we arrived he greeted us as warmly as usual, thanked us for getting the things, and said he would not need anything more. He said he is sure he will be all right tomorrow. It looked to me like he has lost weight since I last saw him, and he said yes, he has lost a few pounds but weighs what the doctor thinks he should.

Even though it has been a month since he moved, he said

he is still tired from moving and will continue to take things easy for a while longer. We had already noticed that a number of boxes sat around, still packed.

Yet, in spite of his weariness and illness, he was as talkative as ever, making funny remarks. Then he became serious and, turning to his niece, said, "Now that I'm settled here, I want to tell you again where certain things are." He did this when he moved into the Home but seemed to want to do it again. He pointed out a file cabinet by his desk and told her what is in each drawer. He added that the key for it is on the ring with his other keys.

"I know I've told you this before," he continued, "but I want to say it again. About my funeral. I want just a graveside service, no flowers. In lieu of flowers, I would like any donations to go to the organization for cancer research." He then told her again the name of his undertaker and that a marker is ready, except for the date of his death, on a plot beside his wife's grave. He emphasized that he does not want an expensive casket. He said, "If Charles Lindbergh, a national hero, could be buried in a cheap pine box, I don't see why I can't."

His niece said to him, as most people do when old people speak of death and burial, "Oh, it will be a long time before we will have to see to that."

"Maybe so," he replied, "but there is one thing I insist on. I do not want the casket opened at any time. I don't want people staring at me when I cannot stare back." We all laughed and spoke of lighter things. But his niece and I agreed after we left that he looked terribly pale.

A *time of partings*. Mr. Brown is dead. He died Thursday at 7 A.M. His death was rather sudden.

Wednesday afternoon I had finished packing to move except for the suitcases of clothes I would need for the month's visit with my daughter in another state. Needless to say, I was physically exhausted and burdened with that feeling of hanging in mid-air that comes when one relinquishes one habitat and has not yet put feet down in a new one. I had stretched out on the bed for a short nap and then planned to get up and dress. My family was getting together for a good-bye dinner for me at an elite restaurant at six o'clock. (I'd had my last meal in the Home and was looking forward to not ever again having to eat another poor meal in the noisy dining room.)

Not more than fifteen minutes elapsed before the phone rang. It was Mr. Brown. He was breathing with difficulty and hardly able to talk. He asked me to call his doctor and come over as quickly as I could. He had not been able to get in touch with either his niece or nephew. I got the doctor immediately.

I dressed quickly and was at his apartment in a few minutes. When I arrived he was lying on the bed and gasping for breath. The doctor called me back saying an ambulance was on the way to take him to the hospital. Mr. Brown could not tell me—in fact, he seemed not to know—what the trouble was. I assumed it was his heart. The ambulance arrived shortly with three men who went to work with first aid treatment. His breathing came easier with oxygen. Before they were ready to leave I got in touch with his niece, who had just gotten home. She said she would be right over (she lives less than a mile away) and go with me to the hospital.

Just as the ambulance crew was ready to leave, I asked one of them if he knew what the trouble was. He said it seemed Mr. Brown had suffered a loss of blood, but they did not know how. He would be given a transfusion as soon as he reached the hospital. I was told to come to Emergency when I got there. Mr. Brown was unconscious when they went out. I left the front door open for his niece to come in and went to the bedroom. It was then I saw the blood.

There was blood on the bed which couldn't be seen till he had been moved. I did not know where it came from. I went around the far side of the bed to get his watch on the table by the bed and saw a large, dark, wet place on the floor. At first I could not take it in. It looked like a pitcher of tomato juice had been poured on the carpet. But it was blood—Mr. Brown's blood.

I went into the bathroom. In the lavatory was a bath towel soaked with blood. Mr. Brown was bleeding his life away.

The niece arrived and we went to the hospital. We had not yet been able to get the nephew. He had left his office and had not reached home.

Mr. Brown was in Intensive Care, being given a transfusion.

The doctor was there. We sat in the room down the hall reserved for family. At long last the doctor came out. He said Mr. Brown's blood pressure was very low, he was in a critical condition, there was every indication of blood loss, and he was puzzled. He wanted me to describe how things were when I arrived. It did not seem at that point that it was heart failure. As soon as I told him about the blood he said that explained it. Mr. Brown had had for some time a condition known as diverticulosis, little pockets in the intestines. After one reaches eighty there is more danger these pockets may break open and an artery may rupture, causing hemorrhaging. He also thought Mr. Brown may have developed a stomach ulcer.

They let us go in and speak to him. He recognized us but seemed very weak. They were able to get his blood pressure up a little. They could not stop the internal bleeding and told us there was nothing that could be done. Early next morning he had two cardiac arrests. When they called his nephew in at seven o'clock to say Mr. Brown had just died, we were not surprised. But I was utterly smitten. Mr. Brown was like a brother to me.

The funeral, a simple graveside service, was conducted at the cemetery where his wife is buried, about thirty miles south of here. Many friends came from the town where he had lived.

Always there comes the let-down. Then come the comforting thoughts: it was good he did not have a long, lingering illness. He had a dread, as most of us do, of becoming helpless and confined to a wheel chair or being bedridden. Yes, he would have wanted to go quickly. But the fact remains, he is gone.

Then come the questions or non-comforting thoughts: too bad he did not have longer in his new set-up; too bad he had changed his place of living because the atmosphere at the Home depressed him; too bad he missed the trip to the mountains he and Mr. Timmons had planned for next week.

The suddenness of it is like a whiplash to me. Just as I was facing moving, he died. In my grief for him, I had to change plane tickets and plans. Moving and his death complicated one another. I feel numb.

The morning after his death I returned to the Home with my daughter to get my things. I sat awhile out in the hall to talk to some friends. My friends were most thoughtful and comforting that morning. They did not have much to say, which I thought was very considerate. They were shocked, they were sad. We all cried a bit.

My parting with them was genuinely sad. I hate to leave them—and would take them with me if I could, for I do not think I will ever come back, not even to visit.

Revival of
My Spirit

Afterthoughts

I have arrived again. Perhaps I should say I have escaped. In any case, I have come to a small retirement home of thirty residents, with a nursing home nearby. Near the ocean, this Home is a one-storied building nestled among many trees—some tropical, others trailing Spanish moss. At times the ocean breeze almost lulls me into euphoria.

Nobody asks, "Do you like it here?" Sometimes I think that would be like asking, "Do you like windows in your house?" I do. Of course, I thought I would like the place I just left, but after only three weeks there I knew I did not, could not like it. I have waited eight weeks here before writing any impressions. I love it.

It is not just that the Home is near the sea that makes me love it. The emotional atmosphere which pervades all aspects of the place is what would make it desirable no matter where it was located.

Beginning with the Administrator and down through all levels of work, every employee is courteous, considerate, and concerned about residents' needs. The morning I moved in, the supervisor of maid service and the maid who would clean my apartment came to see me together. They told me what to expect, chatted about how things are run, and gave me names of others in various capacities. The maid cleans the entire apartment each week and does it thoroughly.

Prior to my moving in, all my dealings were with the young woman in charge of the apartments. A very warm, pleasing person, she made me feel at ease and worthy of courtesy. She said to feel free to call her at any time. After a few days the Administrator of both the retirement home and the nursing home called on me in my apartment. He sat down and, in an unhurried manner, asked if everything was all right and if I needed anything. There were a few things, such as a replacement for a bathroom fixture. He looked at it, surveyed the rest of the apartment, made a list, and assured me all would be taken care of in the near future. It was. It is a good feeling to know you don't have to wait a long time—maybe forever—to get repairs.

Apartments for residents are in buildings of four each. Each two apartments have one entrance, a common porch, and a small yard for each apartment. Many people plant flowers to beautify their yards. With this arrangement, I see my neighbor occasionally but am not faced with a crowd of two hundred people daily in the hall or the dining room. It is good to have one person across the entryway. We keep in touch, and whoever gets out first brings in both papers.

I have an intercom by my bed and an emergency bell in my bathroom. Both connect with the nursing home, where a doctor and a nurse are on call around the clock.

The same kitchen serves both apartment residents and nursing home patients. Nursing home patients who are able, some in wheelchairs, go to a large dining room to eat. Apartment residents eat in a large club room which is also used for bridge parties and other social events. We eat four at a table, as at the other home, but these tables are larger.

One advantage regarding the food itself is that we can eat in the dining room as often as we wish or not at all. We pay only for what we eat. It's much more satisfactory than having to pay for two meals all the time. Many people do not wish to eat with others all the time, but it is good to know we can if we wish.

The food is better than where I was, although there is only one choice for each meal. Sometimes it is not what I would choose, but that could be true even if there were three choices. Anyone who eats here all the time has a well-balanced diet. We are permitted one substitute: fruit instead of the planned dessert. The food is not gourmet, but it is good.

I suffered a state of inertia right after moving in here similar to the one I had right after moving into the other Home. Both times I was physically exhausted from moving. No matter how near or how far you move, how little or much you have to pack and unpack, moving is a change. And change, however good or ill, causes certain stress. Small things, such as getting up on a different side of the bed or remembering on which side of the lavatory the toothbrush holder is placed, take a bit of getting used to.

However, there is this difference in the two moves for me: my lapse of energy in the first instance was increased by my disappointment accompanied by my struggle to overcome it and adjust to the new way of living. I made myself get up earlier, dress before eating, and go to the dining room for breakfast. After two months I came to my senses, slept late because I often read in bed until after midnight, and fixed my own breakfast. Even so, there I always had a feeling of being tied, held in a vise, with all physical movements restricted. Any ambition I had wilted on the vine.

My reaction after settling in here was positive. I was exhausted physically as before, but at the same time I was almost overcome by a sense of release and gladness that I was here. The atmosphere here is such that I can gradually drift into the stream of things, casually and without effort. Neighbors come to call, I meet new people in the club room. Often in late afternoon, after the sun goes down, two, three, or four of us go for a short walk. Some can walk a little further than others. We go or not, as we wish. No feeling exists that you must walk or that you should walk as rapidly as possible with vim and vigor, as if trying to show your age hasn't gotten you yet. No one creeps along walls, holding a hand against them or the tops of chairs trying to show that you do not yet need a stick. No eyes assess you from chairs in the lobby and in the dining room, no one peers from high windows at people getting in and out of their cars.

People here speak frankly of their limitations, without complaint. An attitude of acceptance and sympathy is prevalent, though people do not dwell on their ailments. You know that one has mild arthritis, another very severe, as my neighbor on the right who just can walk enough around her apartment to manage and never goes outside for a walk. One has Parkinson's of a mild sort, and another has the severe kind. Some people are in very good shape and have come here because they no longer wish to live alone.

Those here have very much the same background as the other place: intelligent, well educated, used to an affluent lifestyle, many still drive a car. There is no snobbishness, no formidable cliques, no asking "Will you introduce me to the right people?" Everybody is "right people." I feel comfortable and enjoy being with them.

Gradually the vine of my ambition is beginning to turn a little green. There is no pressure here about anything. It is so good not to receive memos, not to have to decide whether or not I will fill out the next questionnaire. When necessary we receive information. The only regular things we receive are our monthly bills and a copy of the week's menu in our mailbox each Monday morning. We can know in advance when we want to go to the dining room.

Even though I want to forget my experience of the last year-and-a-half, I can't. Most of all I miss Mr. Brown. No friend can take his place. Our friendship lasted all our lives.

Now, I have a new friend next door. She came over to speak to me and welcome me the day I moved in. From each to the other sparked that indefinable something called friendship.

She is a victim—and victim truly describes it—of Parkinson's disease. She does not shake much when under the effects of her medication but often has to leave it off for awhile because of side effects. Then she becomes very weak. If that were not enough, she has an invalid husband in the nursing home nearby. He has been there five years because of a stroke. He speaks very little and has to be fed with a tube. As far as his body is concerned he is a vegetable. Every day after breakfast she goes to the nursing home and sits with him until lunch, which she has in the club room, and then goes back to sit for about two hours. She returns to the apartment quite exhausted and rests the remainder of the day. She is very thin, still a very pretty person, with snow white hair and beautiful, soft brown eyes that speak of something deep within. Her eyes sparkle silently, saying, "I am undefeated."

She reads to her husband and talks to him, and he seems to communicate to her a good deal of what he wants. He can do nothing whatever for himself.

One day I went in to see him. His wife explained who I was. Only his eyes moved, bright blue eyes that also sparkle. He seemed to be saying to me, "I need you, too. I'm glad you and Martha are friends." Love and understanding without words.

Final Musings. We older people need each other. We understand as no one younger really can what it means for your body to fail you by degrees as days and years go by. Sometimes it fails you suddenly. You're never quite ready.

All my life until I was in my eighties I thought of growing old as a gradual process that would bring a slow yielding to the inevitable. I thought I would develop a sense of peace, relief from work, and most responsibility. I envisioned myself sitting on the porch and rocking, doing just what came naturally as nature had her way with me. However, aging does not happen that way. First, depletion takes a sudden dip, then we remain on a kind of plateau for a short or even a long period, then another dip. As for peace, there is no peace or relief when it comes to feeling. The pain of love becomes more intense, along with the joy.

Being human is not easy. Growing old is not easy. If we could really grasp what it is like to be old, *very old*, we might be better able to cope with the limitations of aging, but earlier in life we rather shrink from thinking about growing old, like we don't think much about our own deaths. We plan for aging in some ways, such as saving money or buying health insurance, but how do we build our emotional stockpiles to face our own old age?

The future does not lie in the hands of those of us who are soon to leave this world. Yet are there not a few gems of wisdom about aging that we can bestow on those who follow us so that they may better understand the old ones in their midst and become better able to plan for their own future?

In order to be better prepared for their own old age, I suggest to those coming along that they have more association with old people. Much can be learned from them. True, associations with the old are often not stimulating or interesting and can be boring and difficult. One needs to be patient with the old somewhat in the same manner that we must be patient with the very young—with this difference: the child is striving, but the old person is subsiding. The very nature of the infant is to progress as fast as possible, while the urge of the old person is to let go as slowly and reluctantly as possible. As aging advances and speech, hearing, eyesight, and the ability to move freely begin to lessen, one still retains the memory of things past. A character has developed, a unique personality. Ultimate desires linger, wounds life has inflicted still hurt, good and happy experiences are cherished. However feeble we old ones become, we carry a lot of baggage.

Perhaps the most important thing I have discovered as I've grown old is that the Spirit—that which is me, that which is you—remains the same throughout life. The realization of that becomes stronger in me every day I live. I am the very same Me I was when I took my first breath and let forth my first cry. I am the same Me who ran and played with childhood's joy and was hurt by adults who did not understand. I am the Me who was a restless teenager puzzling about life and love. I am the Me who was a young mother struggling to nurture her children. I am the grandmother enjoying her grandchildren's infancies and the old grandmother leaning on the stalwart arms of their generation. I am the very same Me as the babe I was born—plus eighty-five years of living!

I have not completely deciphered the code of life. But I have come to know deeply the truth Dag Hammarskjöld spoke in *Markings*:

I don't know Who—or what—put the question. I don't know
when it was put. I don't even remember answering. But at some
moment I did answer *Yes* to Someone—or Something—and
from that hour I was certain that existence is meaningful and
that, therefore, my life, in self-surrender, had a goal. (Dag Hammarskjöld, *Markings* [New York: Alfred A. Knopf, 1966], p. 201)

To say *Yes* to life is at one and the same time to say *Yes* to
one's Spirit. If my Spirit says *Yes* to life, how can it say anything but
Yes to death?